l

Illustrated Reviews: Anatomy

Lippincott® Illustrated Reviews: Anatomy

Kelly M. Harrell, PhD, MPT
Assistant Professor
Department of Anatomy and Cell Biology
Brody School of Medicine at East Carolina University
Greenville, North Carolina

Ronald Dudek, PhD
Professor Emeritus
Department of Anatomy & Cell Biology
Brody School of Medicine at East Carolina University
Greenville, North Carolina

Wolters Kluwer

Philadelphia • Baltimore • New York • London
Buenos Aires • Hong Kong • Sydney • Tokyo

Acquisitions Editor: Crystal Taylor
Product Development Editor: Kelly Horvath/Andrea Vosburgh
Editorial Coordinator: Jeremiah Kiely
Editorial Assistant: Brooks Phelps
Marketing Manager: Phyllis Hitner
Production Project Manager: Marian Bellus
Design Coordinator: Steve Druding
Manufacturing Coordinator: Margie Orzech
Prepress Vendor: S4Carlisle Publishing Services

9 8 7 6 5 4 3 2 1

Printed in China

Library of Congress Cataloging-in-Publication Data

Names: Harrell, Kelly, author. | Dudek, Ronald W., 1950- author.
Title: Anatomy / Kelly Harrell, Ronald Dudek.
Other titles: Lippincott's illustrated reviews.
Description: Philadelphia: Wolters Kluwer, [2019] | Series: Lippincott illustrated reviews | Includes bibliographical references.
Identifiers: LCCN 2018042670 | ISBN 9781496317902
Subjects: | MESH: Anatomy | Outlines
Classification: LCC QP34.5 | NLM QS 18.2 | DDC 612—dc23 LC record available at https://lccn.loc.gov/2018042670

shop.lww.com

CCS1018

Dedication

To my Fox and Flower—Knox and Lily,
who inspire me every day to be the best version of myself.
I am forever grateful for the love and laughter you bring to my life.
— Kelly M. Harrell

Acknowledgments

When opportunity comes knocking, you open the door and let it in.

Over 4 years ago, I was asked to come on board to what would be one of the richest learning experiences of my professional life. At the time, the LIR series was missing a vital component—anatomic sciences—that needed to be filled to complete the set. The LIR team reached out to veteran author Ron Dudek to spearhead the task of putting together an integrated embryology, gross anatomy, and histology text. A few days later, I, a lowly assistant professor of anatomy, opened an email from Dr. Dudek that invited me to join as a coauthor. This gracious offer was quickly met with excitement as I formulated my response. With little thought of the time and energy it may require, I said "yes," eager to put my stamp on something of significance in anatomy education.

During the early planning phases, I quickly learned that I would need to rely on my colleagues and students for contributions, whether in the form of radiologic images, consulting, or time spent assisting in dissection. We were assembling a team, and without that team, *LIR Anatomy* would not exist in such a well-rounded, aesthetically pleasing form.

First and foremost, Ron and I would like to acknowledge the anatomic donors and their families for the generous bequeathal of their own or their loved ones' remains. We recognize and honor the ultimate gift, that is, donating one's body for the purposes of educating future health care providers. We are eternally grateful.

Without the leadership of a dedicated and patient development team, *LIR Anatomy* may have faded into the sunset. Crystal Taylor, thank you for trusting Ron and me to create an educational product that upholds the quality of the LIR name. I applaud and appreciate your ability to remain flexible yet firm in your leadership role as Senior Acquisitions Editor, allowing *LIR Anatomy* to come to fruition organically over the past 4 years. I also want to thank you for choosing Kelly Horvath as the freelance Development Editor on this project. I knew, when I signed on, that I would gain a publication, but I never imagined that I would also gain a lifelong colleague and friend in Kelly. Kelly, thank you for your honesty, hard work, countless phone meetings, vivid storytelling, constant support, and friendship. You kept me sane and confident through the past 2 years, and I am so very grateful to be on this team with you.

I also thank the other members of the Wolters Kluwer team who worked behind the scenes to help turn this project into a book. They include Andrea Vosburgh, Internal Development Editor; Jeremiah Kiely, Editorial Coordinator; and Marian Bellus, Production Project Manager. A special thank-you must go to Art Director Jen Clements, who worked miracles to turn our artistic vision into reality. She went above and beyond, putting lots of long hours as well as diligence and care into the art program.

I would like to recognize the clinicians and educators who provided valuable radiologic images and consulting to ensure that the clinical application text and figures were accurate and informative—specifically, interventional and diagnostic radiologists Dr. Michael Berry, Dr. Gregory Lewis, and Dr. Douglas Shusterman (Eastern Radiology, Greenville, NC) and Dr. Michael Meuse (Carolina HealthCare System, Charlotte, NC). Your conscientious contributions to the radiologic components of *LIR Anatomy* are very much appreciated.

I would also like to thank Dr. Robert Hartman, Clinical Assitant Professor of Pediatrics at the Brody School of Medicine for providing the beautiful ultrasound images of pediatric heart defects.

Thank you to the medical and allied health students who took pride and time in preparing clean, complete dissections (Chapters 4 and 7) and were actively involved in developing practice questions (Chapters 8 and 9). Across multiple disciplines, I'd like to thank a small group of students, many of whom have now graduated and moved on to their professional careers. Thank you Dr. Jinal Desai and Dr. Dan-Thanh Nguyen (MD) for your creative and engaging clinical vignette–style practice questions. For assistance with dissections, I'd like to thank my friend and colleague, Dr. Emily Askew; Dr. Amalia Kondyles, Dr. Brandon Kovash, and Dr. Marisa Lee (DPT); Richard Khang; Dr. Samantha Sellers (PhD); and Dr. Asem Rahman (MD). I would also like to acknowledge and thank future-doctor Gabrielle Kattan, for lending her hand modeling skills to Chapter 7.

We also recognize and thank the Brody School of Medicine and the University of California San Francisco School of Medicine for permission to use histology light micrographs from each institution's slide collections.

To Dr. M. Alex Meredith (Medical College of Virginia, Richmond, VA), thank you for sharing your artistic depiction of an area so many learners (and teachers) struggle to imagine and explain—the pterygopalatine fossa. Your willingness to contribute your art and vision of this space has better informed not only *LIR Anatomy* but also countless learners who have passed through our classrooms and laboratories.

Thank you to my parents for their love and encouragement through this process and life in general. You raised me in a nurturing environment, where I was taught to seize my moment, and that approach to life continues to serve me well. Thank you for instilling in me confidence, work ethic, and a love for learning. Those traits have turned this vision into a reality.

Finally, I would like to acknowledge the unyielding support of my husband, Danny. Over the course of coauthoring and designing *LIR Anatomy*, we grew our family from just the two of us to a family of four. Danny, without your encouragement and love, the idea of writing a book while working full time and raising two small children would have seemed impossible. You helped me believe it was possible, and I am forever grateful for your role in the whole process.

Preface

In all living forms, structure dictates function. Take the human skeleton, for example—a bony core that serves as a mobile, yet protective scaffold onto which our tissues are successively layered, producing our adaptable, fluid bodies. In each unique tissue, intricate cells and fibers flow together to fill a role—movement, transport, protection, stability, nutrition, procreation, storage, intelligence, sensation, life, and, ultimately, death.

From a young age, I was in awe of the way these structures coexist and function together within a single vessel. Even in light of variation or anomaly, the human body almost always finds a way to grow, evolve, and accommodate within its own environment. It is truly a marvel to be studied and celebrated.

The study of anatomy is a journey across the microscopic landscape of cells and tissues into the macroscopic topography of organ systems. Much like the estuaries of eastern North Carolina, anatomy comprises small structures merging to form larger structures and functioning within a physiologic ebb and flow. Just as small creeks fill grooves carved into earth and merge to form tributaries and rivers, histologic examination of human tissue shows how cells and microscopic structures merge and coordinate as larger organs. Just as rivers expand into sounds and eventually flow out to sea, human organs integrate as body systems. The estuary represents the place where the river meets the sea, an intersection seen in the study of the human body where histology meets gross anatomy.

This intersection of histology and gross anatomy is underpinned by embryology. These three streams of anatomic science converge in a novel way in the first edition of *LIR Anatomy* to better elucidate the structural and functional details of the human body. So unique in its layout, *LIR Anatomy* regionally integrates embryology, gross anatomy, and histology together in a single source to highlight the important relationships that exist across these topics.

Purpose: Since its inception, *LIR Anatomy* has been designed to precipitate those "ah-ha" moments that occur when learners follow related topics along a continuum of time and space. As the puzzle begins to come together, learners build on their understanding in a more integrative fashion. Studies show that thoughtful integration of topics leads to deeper learning and retention. This theory underpins the shift of many medical schools from traditional to integrated curricula. *LIR Anatomy* augments this approach to learning with writing that is engaging, well-organized, and informative.

Audience: *LIR Anatomy* is written as a detailed review text with medical students in mind. From day 1 of medical school, students must integrate basic science topics and organize them to promote learning and retention. In the short term, medical students are most concerned with performance on licensing exams. The integration of all three anatomic science topics—embryology, gross anatomy, and histology—provides learners with a valuable resource for immediate exam preparation and future clinical reference.

Although succinct enough for review purposes, *LIR Anatomy* is comprehensive in its treatment of the anatomic science triumvirate, making it an appropriate primary text in allied health programs that incorporate these topics.

Art: *LIR Anatomy* art brings the text to life with interactive figures that walk the reader through processes and concepts in a systematic, comprehensible manner. Images are further invigorated with strategically placed tips and mnemonics in the series' signature dialogue bubbles. Figures also include directional labels to assist readers in orientation to structures on a two-dimensional page. Clear, crisp histologic images display unique tissue characteristics across systems, while color-coded schematic embryologic figures take readers through the step-wise process of human development.

The hallmark of *LIR Anatomy* art is its cadaveric specimens, which were carefully dissected just for this book, photographed, and then digitally enhanced to present realistic yet idealized views of the inside of the human body. Coloring, labeling, and "narration" highlight the arrangement of gross anatomic structures in a more three-dimensional format.

Format: *LIR Anatomy* is designed to be both narrative and concise. The outline-format chapters are organized by anatomic region and further subdivided into easy-to-digest sections. Each chapter follows a similar progression, with embryology presented up front, followed by gross anatomy and histology. This approach allows readers to integrate topics, while continuing to support the traditional, regional method common to the study of anatomic sciences. This two-pronged system allows for easy adoption across different curricular models.

Features: *LIR Anatomy* incorporates a variety of features to facilitate integrative learning within a clinical context.

- **Clinical applications (blue boxes):** Learning anatomy out of context is like fishing without a lure—you aren't going to catch anything! Each chapter provides high-yield clinical anatomy applications in blue boxes that give readers insight into the utility of the content in practice. Additionally, clinical applications illustrate how important a solid foundational knowledge in the anatomic sciences is in the diagnosis of common pathologies and injuries.
- **Knowledge morsels (green boxes):** Whether it is a helpful mnemonic or a stand-out structural or functional detail, green boxes are incorporated in each chapter to augment learning. These tidbits of information reinforce and supplement both the main text and the adjacent figures.
- **Dialogue bubbles:** Dialogue bubbles have been added to figures to remind readers of important relationships, further integrate topics, highlight clinically significant information, and provide learners with helpful study tips. As readers process the figures, they can imagine the authors taking a moment to interject and engage in a discussion. Readers should use these memorable dialogues as prompts for further thought and discussion in each chapter.
- **Study questions:** Board-style practice questions on high-yield topics are included at the end of each chapter for self-assessment. These questions are written to address the first three levels of Bloom's taxonomy—knowledge, understanding, and application. Many questions are presented in clinical-vignette style to provide opportunity for learners to practice applying knowledge in a low-stakes environment before sitting for licensing exams.

—Kelly M. Harrell, PhD, MPT

Contents

Anatomy Foundations

1

I. OVERVIEW

A thorough evaluation of the anatomical sciences involves the intersection of three subjects—gross anatomy, embryology, and histology. This review text integrates all three anatomical subjects into a region-based model divided into back, thorax, abdomen, pelvis, upper limb, lower limb, neck, and head and cranial nerves chapters. While maintaining this overall integration within each body region, each chapter is subdivided to cover gross anatomy, embryology, and histology in discrete chunks that help delineate the content. In order to fully understand the content in each chapter, a foundation of anatomical terminology and an overview of organ-system organization are required, as this introductory chapter is designed to provide. Gross anatomy body systems are covered here, while body regions are covered in chapters corresponding to relevant anatomy. Select clinical conditions are interspersed throughout chapters in Clinical Application boxes to connect anatomy to clinical practice. In addition, a brief discussion of radiographic anatomy at the end of this chapter provides learners with basic radiologic terminology to aid in orientation to diagnostic images included throughout the text.

A. Anatomical position

Anatomical position refers to the body position in which an individual is standing upright with the head and toes facing forward, the upper limbs adjacent to the sides of the body with the palms facing forward, and the lower limbs close together with feet parallel (Fig. 1.1).

B. Anatomical planes

Four imaginary planes are used in anatomical descriptions: **median**, **sagittal**, **frontal** (**coronal**), and **transverse (axial) planes** (see Fig. 1.1). The median plane is a vertical plane that passes longitudinally through the midline of the body and divides the body into the right and left halves. The sagittal planes are vertical planes that pass longitudinally through the body parallel to the median plane. The frontal (coronal) planes are vertical planes that pass through the body at right angles to the median plane and divide the body into the front (anterior or ventral) and back (posterior or dorsal) parts. The transverse planes are horizontal planes that pass through the body at right angles to the median plane and divide the body into upper (superior) and lower (inferior) parts.

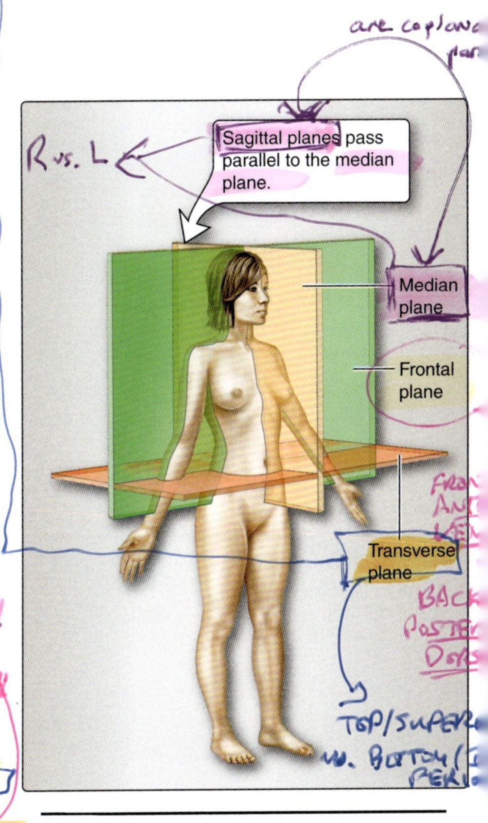

Figure 1.1
Anatomical planes.

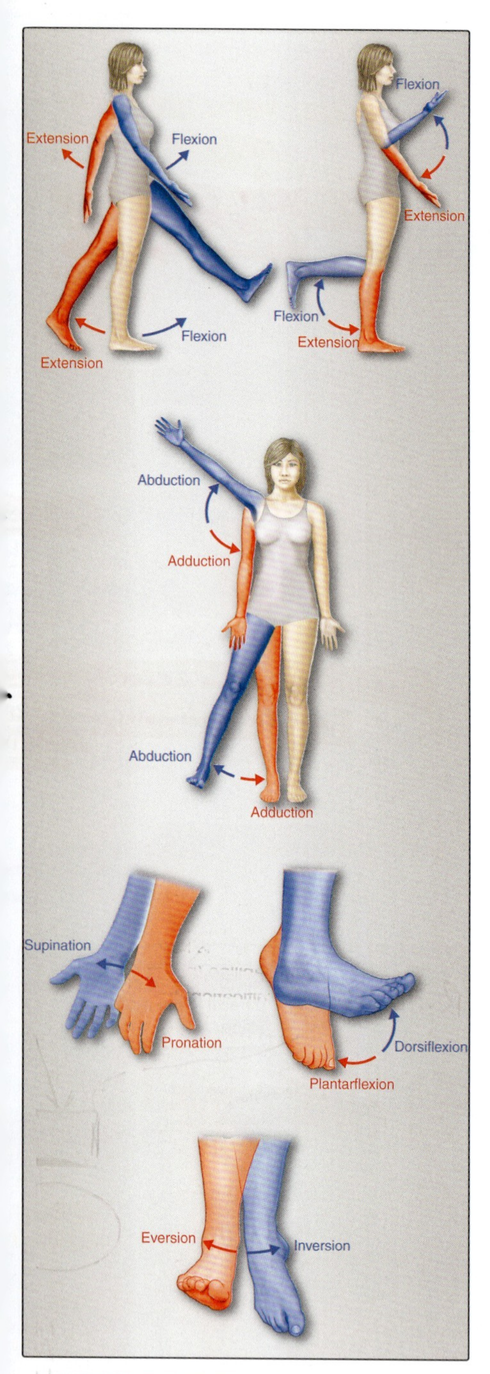

Figure 1.2
Anatomical movements.

Table 1.1: Terms of Relationship

Term	Description
Medial	Refers to a structure nearer to the median plane
Lateral	Refers to a structure farther from the median plane
Proximal	Refers to a structure nearer a limb attachment
Distal	Refers to a structure farther from a limb attachment
Bilateral	Refers to paired structures having right and left members
Unilateral	Refers to unpaired structures that occur only on one side
Ipsilateral	Refers to a structure that occurs on the same side as another structure
Contralateral	Refers to a structure that occurs on the opposite side as another structure

C. Anatomical terms of relationship

The terms *superior* and *cranial* refer to a structure nearer the cranium. The terms *inferior* and *caudal* refer to a structure nearer the foot. The terms *posterior* and *dorsal* refer to the back surface of the body. The terms *anterior* and *ventral* refer to the front surface of the body. [**Note**: In this text, "cranial," "caudal," "dorsal," and "ventral" are used only in the context of embryology.] Other important terms are presented in Table 1.1.

D. Anatomical terms of movement

As shown in Figure 1.2, *flexion* describes a movement that decreases the angle between the bones, whereas *extension* describes a movement that increases the angle between the bones. Except when referring to the digits, *abduction* describes a movement away from the median plane (as in the upper limb moving away from the body), whereas *adduction* describes a movement toward the median plane (as in the upper limb moving toward the body). *Pronation* describes a rotation in the forearm from the anatomical position so that the palm of the hand faces posteriorly, and *supination* describes a rotation in the forearm whereby the pronated hand returns to the anatomical position so that the palm of the hand faces anteriorly. *Dorsiflexion* describes flexion at the ankle joint as in lifting the toes off the ground, and *plantarflexion* describes flexion at the ankle joint as in lifting the heel off the ground. *Eversion* describes a movement of the foot whereby the sole moves away from the median plane, whereas *inversion* describes a movement of the foot whereby the sole of the foot moves toward the median plane. Finally, movements that are unique to the hands and feet, particularly the digits of the hands, are shown in Table 1.2.

II. INTEGUMENTARY SYSTEM

The integumentary system consists of the **skin** and **epidermal derivatives** (or **epidermal appendages**). Skin forms the outer covering of the body and is the largest organ of the body, accounting for 15%–20% of the total body weight. Epidermal derivatives include **sweat** and **sebaceous glands**, **hair** and **hair follicles**, and **nails**.

A. Functions

Collectively, skin and epidermal derivatives regulate body temperature and water loss, provide a nonspecific barrier to external environmental factors (e.g., microorganisms), synthesize vitamin D, absorb ultraviolet

Table 1.2: Terms of Movement of the Hands and Feet

Term	Movement Described
Flexion of the digits	**Fingers move toward the palm, flexing at the MCP and IP joints**
Extension of the digits	**Fingers return from flexion to anatomical position, extending at the MCP and IP joints**
Abduction of the digits	**Fingers spread away from a neutral-positioned third finger (middle finger) or the toes from a neutral-positioned second toe**
Adduction of the digits	**Fingers "un-spread" back toward a neutral-positioned third finger (middle finger) or the toes toward a neutral-positioned second toe**
Opposition of the thumb	**Thumb touches the pad of another finger**
Reposition of the thumb	**Thumb returns from opposition to anatomical position**
Abduction of the thumb	**Thumb moves away from the fingers in the sagittal plane**
Adduction of the thumb	**Thumb moves toward the fingers in the sagittal plane**
Flexion of the thumb	**Thumb moves toward the fingers in the frontal plane**
Extension of the thumb	**Thumb moves away from the fingers in the frontal plane**

IP = interphalangeal, MCP = metacarpophalangeal.

(UV) irradiation, convey sensory information, play a role in antigen presentation, and secrete sweat and sebum.

B. Skin

In general, skin consists of three layers, **outer epidermis**, **middle dermis**, and **deep hypodermis** or **subcutaneous layer**.

1. **Outer epidermis:** The outer epidermis is an epithelial layer classified as a keratinized stratified squamous epithelium. On the basis of the comparative thickness of the epidermis, skin is classified as either **thick skin** (found on palms of the hands or soles of the feet) or **thin skin** (covering the rest of the body), as shown in Figures 1.3 and 1.4.

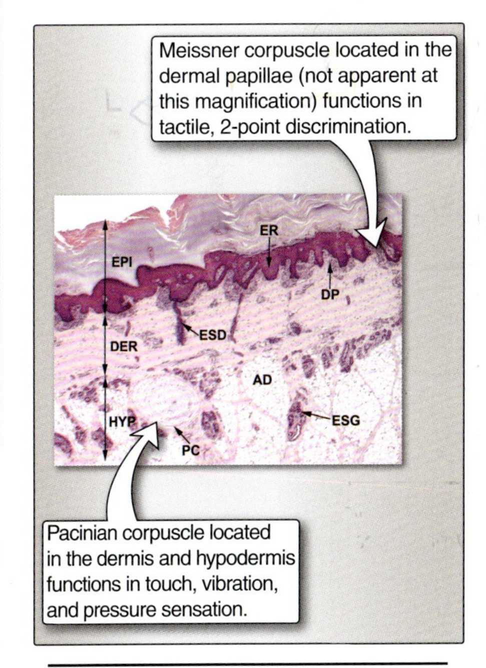

Figure 1.3
Thick skin. AD = adipose tissue, DER = dermis, DP = dermal papillae, EPI = epidermis, ER = epidermal ridge, ESD = eccrine sweat gland duct, ESG = eccrine sweat gland, HYP = hypodermis, PC = Pacinian corpuscle.

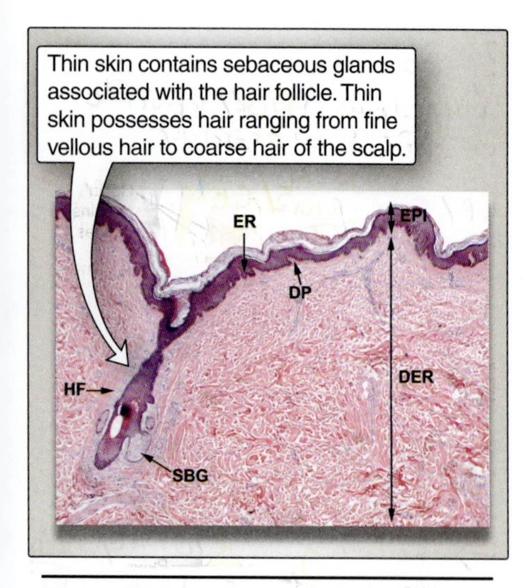

Figure 1.4
Thin skin. DER = dermis, DP = dermal papillae, EPI = epidermis, ER = epidermal ridge, HF = hair follicle, SBG = sebaceous gland.

2. **Dermis**: The junction between the epidermis and dermis is irregular, whereby **epidermal ridges** protrude into the underlying dermis, and **dermal papillae** protrude into the overlying epidermis (see Fig. 1.3). The dermis is composed of the **papillary layer** and **reticular layer**. The superficial papillary layer (i.e., the dermal papillae) consists of loose connective tissue with fibroblasts, types I and III collagen fibers, and thin elastic fibers. The deeper reticular layer consists of dense, irregular connective tissue with fibroblasts, type I collagen, and thick elastic fibers. In addition, skin contains a number of epidermal derivatives (also called **epidermal appendages**): **eccrine** and **apocrine sweat glands**, **sebaceous glands**, **hair follicles** (and **arrector pili muscles**), and **nails**.

C. Epidermal derivatives

1. **Eccrine sweat glands and duct**: These simple, coiled tubular glands are involved in the secretion of **water**, **electrolytes**, **urea**, and **ammonium**. The duct opens onto the skin surface as **sweat pores**. The eccrine sweat glands function in the regulation of body temperature and emotional sweating.
2. **Apocrine sweat glands and duct**: These simple, coiled tubular glands are involved in the secretion of **proteins**, **carbohydrates**, **ammonia**, **lipid**, and **organic compounds**. The duct opens onto the skin surface in the axilla, mons pubis, and anal regions. The apocrine sweat glands function in the production of a malodorous body scent.
3. **Sebaceous glands and duct**: These simple acinar glands are involved in the secretion of **sebum** (i.e., lipid and cell debris). The short duct opens into the upper portion of a hair follicle into the **pilosebaceous canal**. The sebaceous glands function in the lubrication of the skin and play a role in teenage acne.
4. **Hair follicles**: These form as epidermal cells and grow into the underlying dermis during early embryonic development. The deepest part of the hair follicle becomes round-shaped and is called the **hair bulb**. The hair bulbs are invaginated by connective tissue called the **dermal papillae**, which are infiltrated by blood vessels and nerve endings. Epidermal cells within the hair bulb form an area containing **epidermal stem cells** called the **germinal matrix**. The continuous proliferation and differentiation of germinal matrix cells at the tip of the dermal papilla is responsible for the formation and growth of the **hair shaft**, a long, slender filament that extends above the surface of the epidermis.
5. **Nail**: The nail is a translucent plate (called the **nail plate**) of closely compacted **hard keratin** formed by the proliferation and keratinization of epithelial cells within the **nail matrix**. The nail matrix is a V-shaped area located under a fold of skin called the **proximal nail fold**. The only portion of the nail matrix that is grossly visible is the **lunula**, a half moon–shaped whitish area. At the outer edge of the proximal nail fold is the **eponychium** or **cuticle**. The nail rests on top of the nail bed. At the fingertip, the nail and the nail bed fuse to form the **hyponychium**, which protects the nail matrix from bacterial and fungal invasion. The dermis beneath the nail bed is highly vascular, which contributes to the pink color seen through the nail, and is a clinically useful indicator of the degree of oxygenation of blood.

III. SKELETAL SYSTEM

The skeletal system is divided into the **axial skeleton** and the **appendicular skeleton** (Fig. 1.5). The axial skeleton consists of bones of the cranium (or skull), hyoid bone, ribs, sternum, vertebrae, and sacrum. The appendicular skeleton consists of the bones of the upper and lower limbs, shoulder girdle, and pelvic girdle. The skeleton is composed of **cartilage** and **bone**.

A. Cartilage

The three types of cartilage include **hyaline cartilage**, **elastic cartilage**, and **fibrocartilage**.

1. **Hyaline cartilage**: Hyaline cartilage is found in fetal skeletal tissue, epiphyseal growth plates, articular surface of synovial joints, costal cartilages, nasal cartilage, laryngeal cartilage, tracheal cartilage rings, and bronchial cartilage plates. Its main features are **cells**, including **chondrogenic cells**, **chondroblasts**, and **chondrocytes**; a **ground substance**, containing **proteoglycans** (e.g., **aggrecan**, **decorin**, **biglycan**, and **fibromodulin**), **hyaluronan**, **multiadhesive glycoproteins** (e.g., **chondronectin**, **tenascin**), and **water** (**interstitial fluid**); and **fibers**, including **types II**, **VI**, **IX**, **X**, and **XI collagen** (Fig. 1.6).
2. **Elastic cartilage**: Elastic cartilage is found in the pinna of the external ear, external auditory meatus, auditory tube, epiglottis, corniculate cartilage of the larynx, and cuneiform cartilage of the larynx. Its main features are similar to those of hyaline cartilage (Fig. 1.7). However, the distinguishing feature of elastic cartilage is the presence of **elastic fibers** along with **type II collagen fibers**. Elastic cartilage is generally stained with a special stain (i.e., Verhoeff) that colors elastic fibers black.
3. **Fibrocartilage**: Fibrocartilage is found in intervertebral disks, symphysis pubis, articular disks of the temporomandibular and sternoclavicular joints, menisci of the knee joint, and insertion of tendons. Its main features are similar to that of hyaline cartilage (Fig. 1.8). However, the distinguishing features of fibrocartilage include the absence of a perichondrium, more extracellular matrix than cells, and the presence of types I and II collagen fibers.

B. Bone

Bones can be classified according to their shape. **Long bones** are tubular (e.g., humerus), and **short bones** are cuboidal (e.g., bones of the wrist and ankle). **Flat bones** serve a protective function (e.g., bones of the cranium). **Irregular bones** have various shapes (e.g., bones of the face), and **sesamoid bones** form in certain tendons (e.g., patella bone of the knee). Visual inspection of a bone reveals various **bone markings**, created by the attachment of tendons, ligaments, and fascia or by the close proximity of an artery to the bone or where an artery enters the bone, and **bone formations** caused by the passage of a tendon to a joint to improve its leverage. The main features of bone are **cells** (**osteoprogenitor cells**, **osteoblasts**, **osteocytes**, and **osteoclasts**), a **ground substance** (**proteoglycans**, **hyaluronan**, **multiadhesive glycoproteins**, **vitamin K–dependent proteins**, and a **mineral**

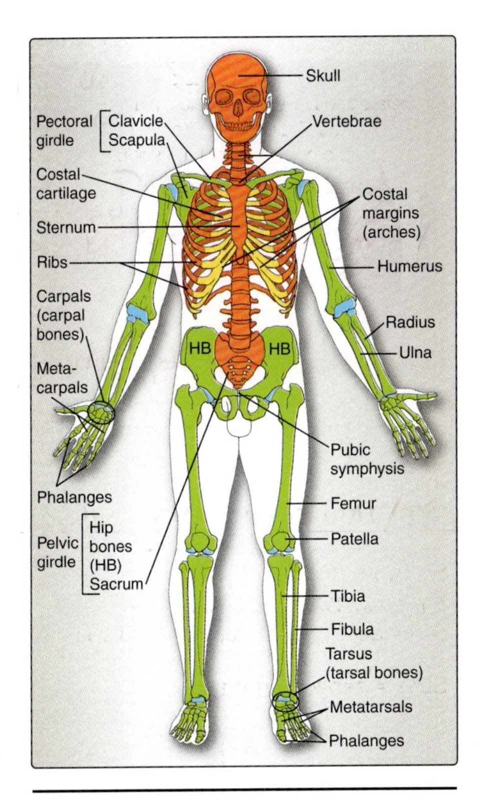

Figure 1.5
Skeletal system comprises the axial skeleton (red) and the appendicular skeleton (green) as well as articular (blue) and costal (yellow) cartilage.

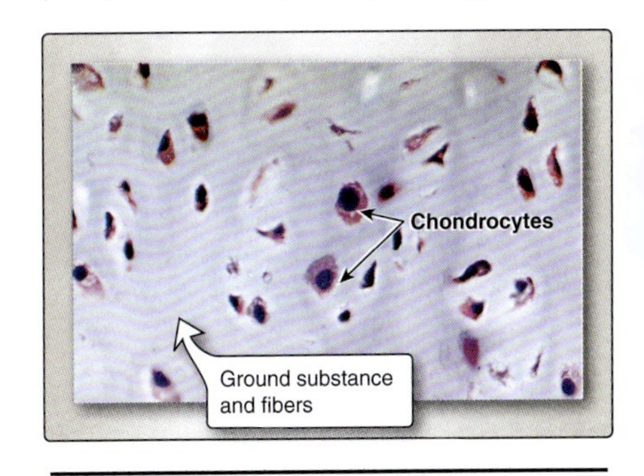

Figure 1.6
Hyaline cartilage.

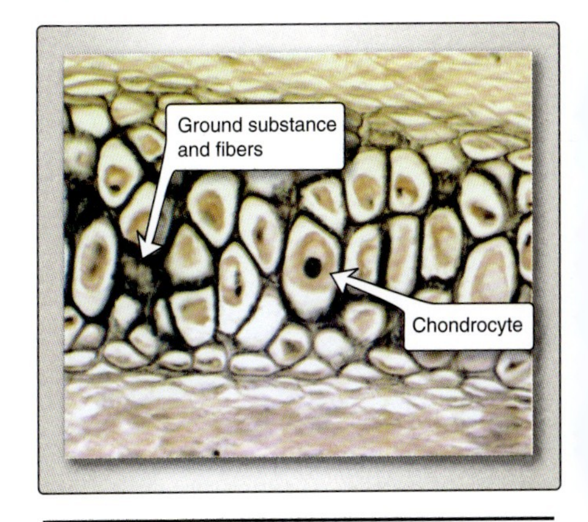

Figure 1.7
Elastic cartilage.

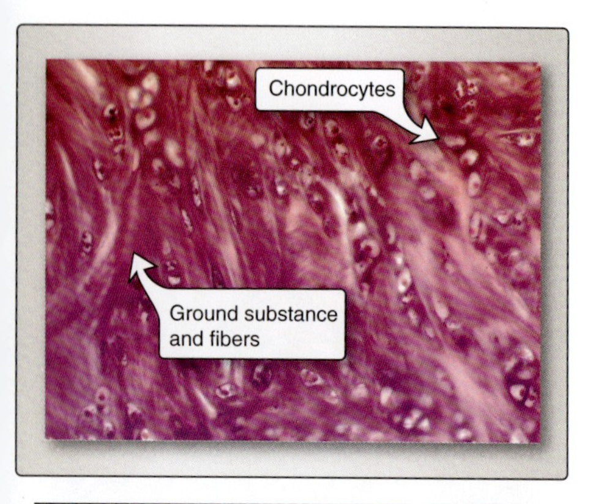

Figure 1.8
Fibrocartilage.

component of **hydroxyapatite crystals** [Ca_{10} $(PO_4)_6$ OH_2]), and **fibers** that include **types I** and **V collagen**.

1. **Lamellar bone**: Comprising virtually all bone in a healthy adult, lamellar bone is therefore sometimes referred to as **mature bone**. (**Woven bone** comprises bone during embryonic development, bone remodeling, and bone repair and is therefore sometimes referred to as **immature bone**.) Lamellar bone (compared with woven bone) is characterized by an ordered arrangement of osteocytes, a reduced amount of ground substance, a regular parallel arrangement of collagen fibers organized into lamellae or layers, and increased mineralization. It is divided into two types: **compact bone** and **spongy bone** (Fig. 1.9).

> Although collagen fibers are oriented in a parallel arrangement within a single lamella, they alternate from lamella to lamella, creating an overall zig-zag appearance.

a. **Compact bone**: As shown in Figure 1.9, compact bone consists predominately of **osteons** (or **Haversian systems**). The osteon is the basic unit of compact bone and consists of an **osteonal** (**Haversian**) **canal** and **perforating** (**Volkmann**) **canals** through

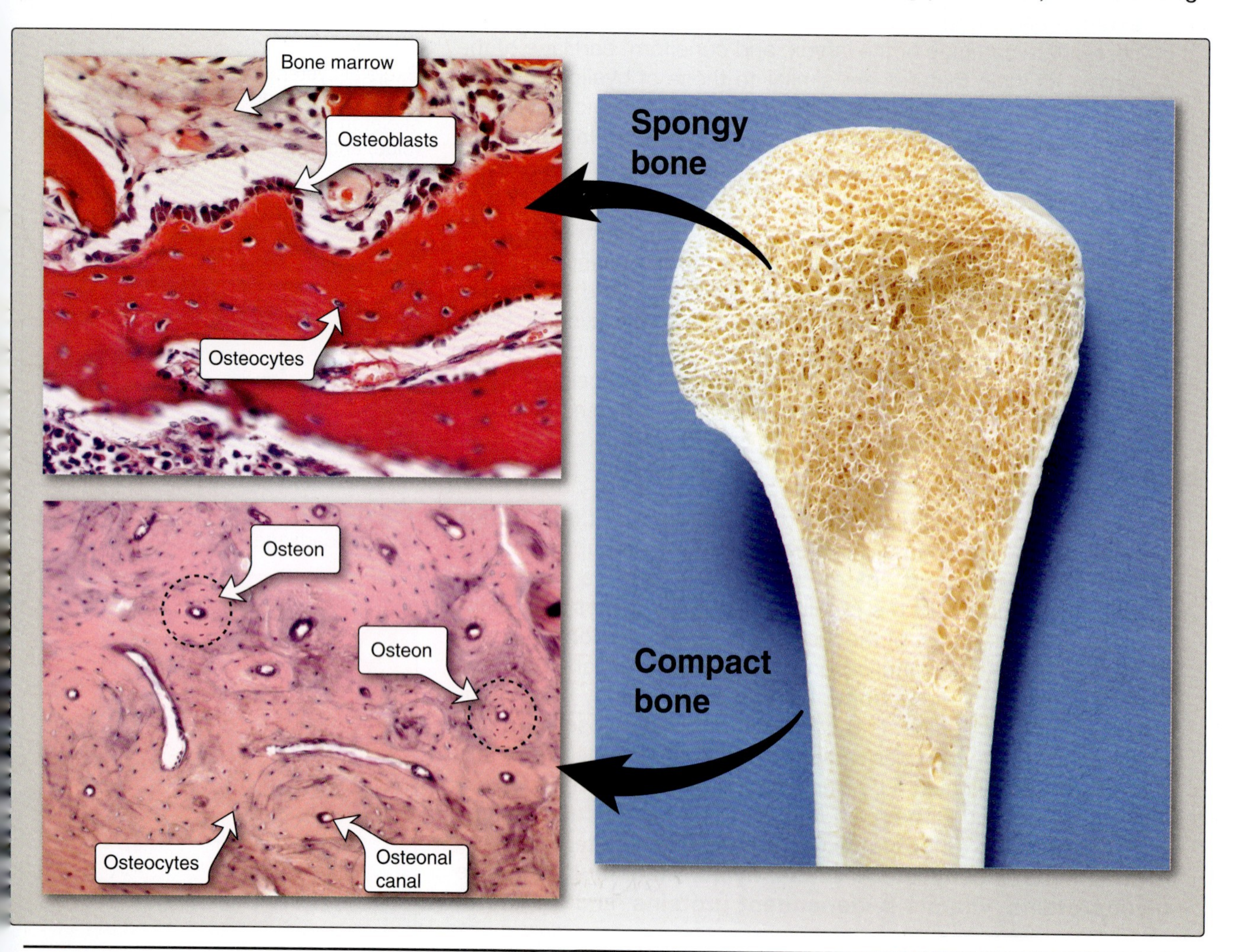

Figure 1.9
Spongy and compact bone.

which blood vessels and nerves travel, **concentric lamellae** (layers) of mineralized extracellular matrix that surround the osteonal canal, **collagen fibers** that are oriented in a parallel arrangement within a single lamella, **osteocytes** whose cell bodies reside in **lacunae** and whose cell processes extend through **canaliculi**, and a **cement line** that surrounds each osteon.

b. Spongy bone: Spongy bone consists predominately of a meshwork of internal struts called **trabeculae** (see Fig. 1.9). The lamellae in spongy bone are arranged in a stacked pattern (i.e., one layer on top of another layer), rather than in the concentric pattern found in the osteon of compact bone.

IV. MUSCULAR SYSTEM

Muscles of the human body comprise three types: **cardiac, smooth, and skeletal** (Fig. 1.10; see also Fig. 3.52A). Cardiac muscle forms the walls of the heart. Cardiac muscle cells are striated but smaller than skeletal

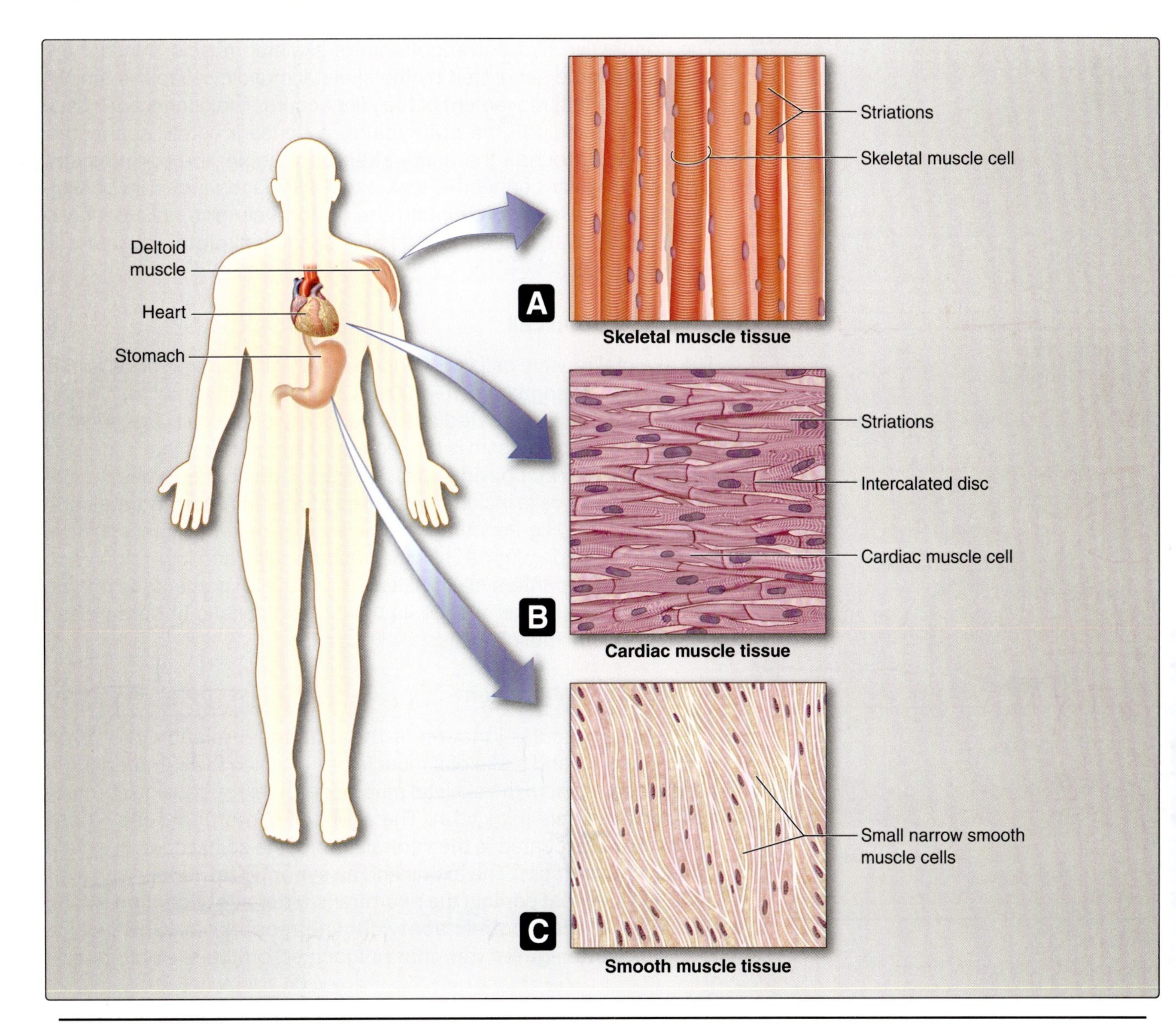

Figure 1.10
Muscle tissue. A, Skeletal muscle. B, Cardiac muscle. C, Smooth muscle.

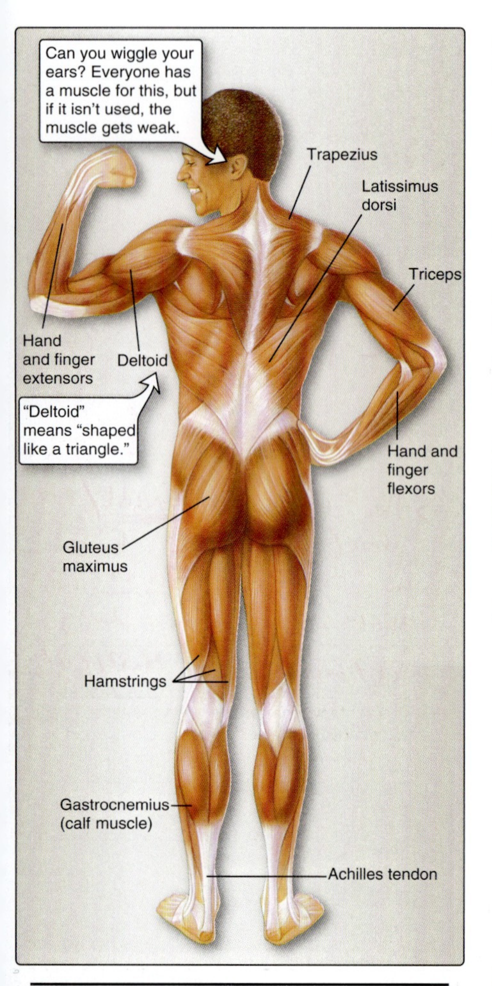

Figure 1.11
Skeletal muscles.

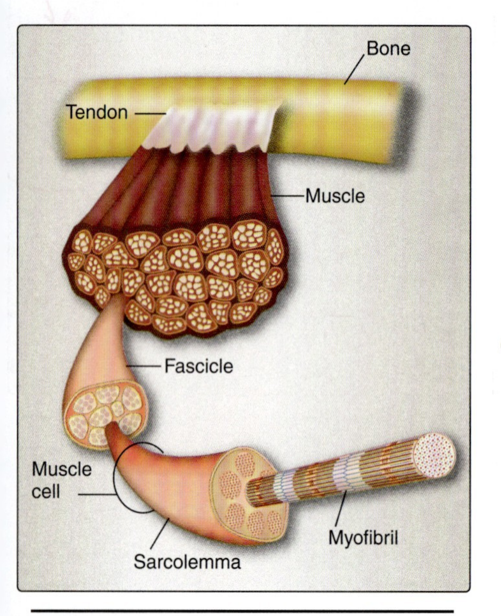

Figure 1.12
Skeletal muscle organization.

muscle cells and have a single nucleus per cell. Smooth muscle is primarily found in the walls of hallow viscera and blood vessels. Smooth muscle cells lack striations, have one nucleus per cell, and are small and narrow in appearance. Cardiac and smooth muscle are detailed in Chapters 3 and 4, respectively.

The gross Skeletal muscle cells are striated and converge to form skeletal muscles of varied shapes and sizes (Fig 1.11). As shown in Table 1.3, skeletal muscles can be described according to their shape. A **skeletal muscle** (e.g., biceps brachii muscle) consists of numerous **fascicles**, which consist of numerous **skeletal muscle cells** (also called **skeletal muscle fibers**). A skeletal muscle cell, in turn, consists of numerous **myofibrils** comprising **thick and thin myofilaments** (Fig. 1.12).

Skeletal muscle → Fascicles → Skeletal muscle cells → Myofibrils → Myofilaments

A. Connective tissue components

The connective tissue components of skeletal muscle transmit the contractile force generated by the skeletal muscle cell to the tendon and bone so that movement of the joint occurs. The connective tissue components include the **epimysium**, a dense irregular connective tissue that surrounds the entire **skeletal muscle**; the **perimysium**, a dense irregular connective tissue that surrounds a bundle of skeletal muscle cells (**fascicle**); and the **endomysium**, a delicate loose connective tissue that surrounds an individual **skeletal muscle cell** (see Fig. 1.12).

B. Skeletal muscle cell

The skeletal muscle cell is cylinder shaped with tapered ends and is ~2–100 mm in length and 10–100 μm in diameter. It is multinucleated with thin, flat nuclei located at the periphery of the cell. As shown in Figure 1.13, its cytoplasm is characterized by striations that consist of the **A band** (**dark**), **I band** (**light)**, and the **Z disc**. The three types of skeletal muscle cells include **type I** (**red**), **type IIa (intermediate**), and **type IIb** (**white**). High-endurance athletes (e.g., marathon runners) have a high percentage of type I skeletal muscle cells, and low-endurance athletes (e.g., sprinters, weightlifters) have a high percentage of type IIb skeletal muscle cells. Type IIa have characteristic of both types I and IIb skeletal muscle cells.

C. Neuromuscular junction

The neuromuscular junction is the junctional relationship of an α-motoneuron and a skeletal muscle cell in which the α-motoneuron transmits a signal to the skeletal muscle cell, thereby causing contraction of the muscle (Fig. 1.14). The axons of **α-motoneurons** whose cell bodies are located in the ventral horn of the spinal cord innervate skeletal muscle cells. The axons end as **synaptic terminals** with synaptic vesicles that contain the neurotransmitter **acetylcholine** (**ACh)**. ACh binds to the **nicotinic acetylcholine receptor** (**nAChR**), which is a **transmitter-gated ion channel** located on the skeletal muscle

Table 1.3: Muscle Shapes

Shape	Muscle Example	
Flat	External oblique muscle of the abdomen	
Pennate	Rectus femoris muscle	
Fusiform	Biceps brachii	
Multiheaded	Triceps brachii	
Convergent	Pectoralis major	
Quadrate	Rectus abdominis	
Circular	Orbicularis oculi	
Multibellied	Gastrocnemius	

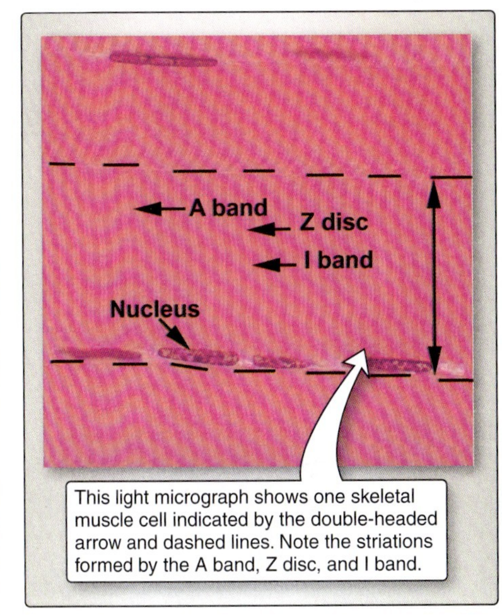

Figure 1.13
Skeletal muscle cell.

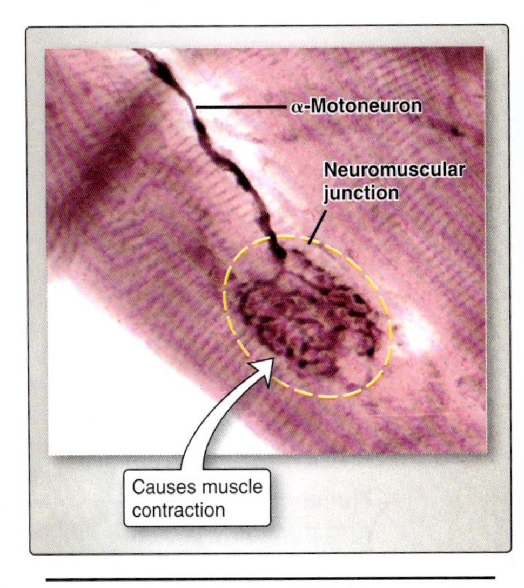

Figure 1.14
Neuromuscular junction.

cell. When ACh binds to nAChR, a "gate" opens and allows **Na^+ influx** into the skeletal muscle cell, causing depolorization.

D. Motor unit

A single axon of an α-motoneuron may innervate 1 to 5 skeletal muscle cells, which forms a **small motor unit**. Or, a single axon of an α-motoneuron may branch and innervate more than 150 skeletal muscle cells, forming a **large motor unit**.

> A motor unit is the **functional contractile unit** of a gross skeletal muscle, not a skeletal muscle cell.

E. Muscle spindle

As shown in Figure 1.15, the muscle spindle is a small, elongated, encapsulated structure distributed throughout a gross skeletal muscle that senses both **dynamic changes in muscle length** and **static muscle length** as well as activating the **myotactic (stretch) reflex** (e.g., knee jerk reflex). It consists of **nuclear bag cells** and **nuclear chain cells** and is innervated by **type Ia sensory neurons (annulo-spiral endings)**, **type II sensory neurons (flower-spray endings)**, and **γ-motoneurons**.

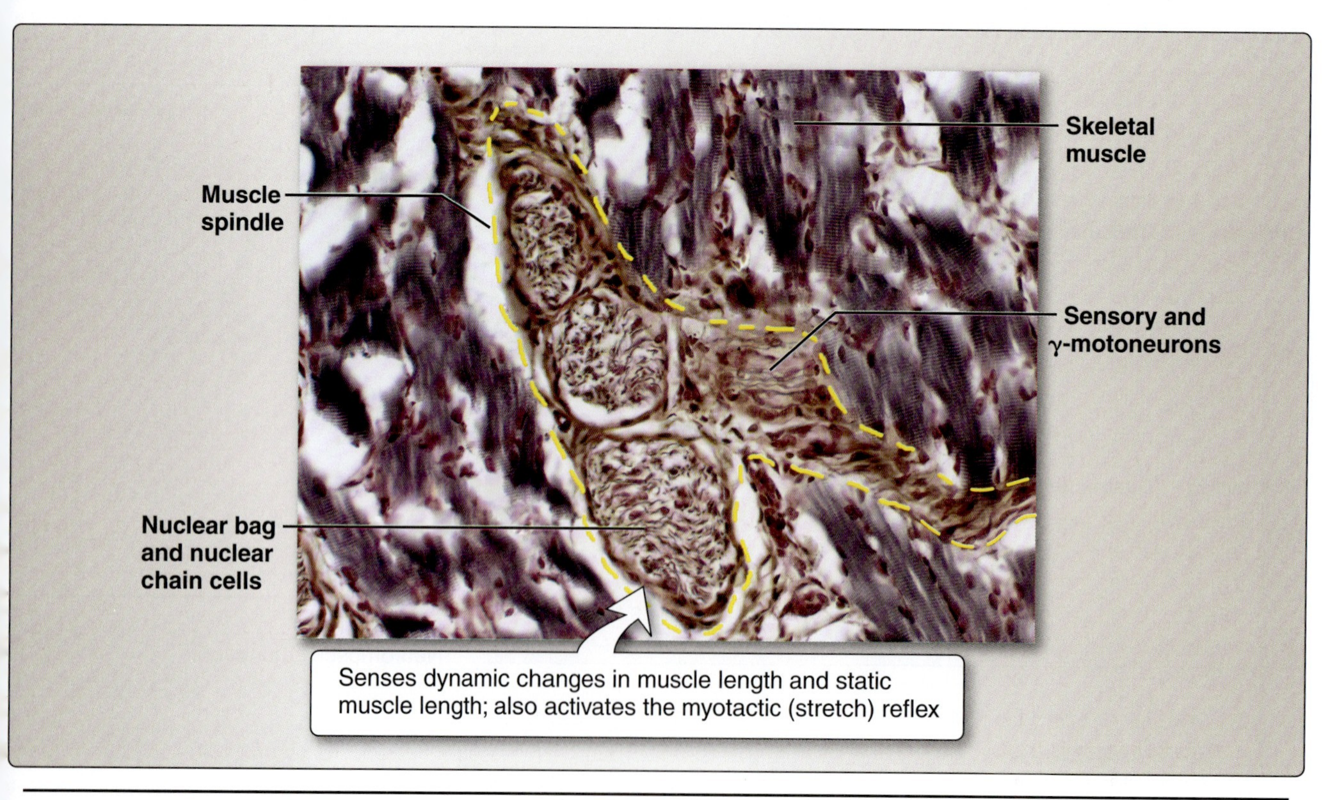

Figure 1.15
Muscle spindle (yellow dashed line).

V. CARDIOVASCULAR SYSTEM

The cardiovascular system consists of the **heart** and **blood vessels** that circulate blood throughout the body (Fig. 1.16).

A. Heart

The heart consists of two muscular pumps that divide the blood circulation into two circuits (Fig. 1.17). In the **pulmonary circulation**, the right ventricle pumps low-oxygen blood into the lungs via the **pulmonary arteries** where the blood is oxygenated and then returned to the left atrium of the heart via the **pulmonary veins**. In the **systemic circulation**, the left ventricle pumps highly oxygenated blood through the **systemic arteries** to distribute oxygen and nutrients throughout the body. Low-oxygen blood is returned to the right atrium of the heart via **systemic veins**.

B. Blood vessels

The three general types of blood vessels are **arteries**, **capillaries**, and **veins**, which distribute blood throughout the body. For a summary of blood vessel types, see Figure 1.20.

> Systemic blood flow follows a particular pathway:
> Elastic arteries → Muscular arteries → Arterioles → Metarterioles → Capillary bed →
> Postcapillary venules → Muscular venules → Collecting venules → Veins of increasing diameter (named veins)

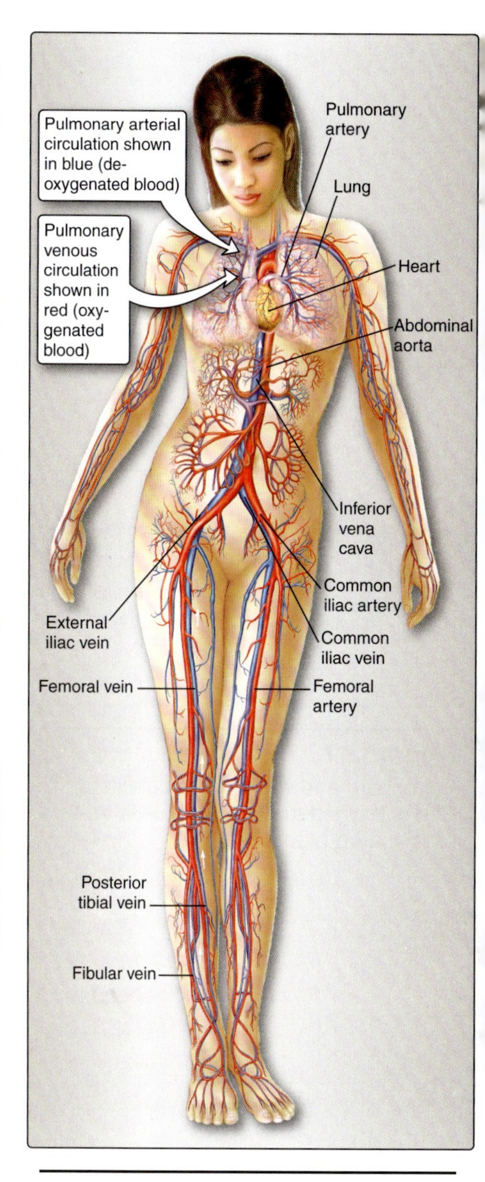

Figure 1.16
Cardiovascular system.

1. **Arteries**: The vascular wall of arteries consists of three concentric layers ("tunics"): **tunica intima**, **tunica media**, and **tunica adventitia** (Fig. 1.18). The tunica intima is the innermost layer and consists of the **endothelium**, **basal lamina**, **subendothelial loose connective tissue**, and an **internal elastic lamina**. The tunica media is the middle layer and consists of **smooth muscle cells**, **type III collagen fibers**, **elastic fibers**, and an **external elastic lamina**. The tunica adventitia is the outermost layer and consists of **fibroblasts**, **type I collagen fibers**, and **scattered elastic fibers**. The tunica adventitia of large arteries contains small blood vessels (**vasa vasorum**), small postganglionic sympathetic nerve bundles (**nervi vascularis**), and small **lymph vessels**. In the circulatory system, elastic arteries gradually transition to large muscular arteries (i.e., no line demarcates them). In the region of transition, the amount of elastic fibers in the tunica media decreases, whereas the amount of smooth muscle whereas the amount of smooth muscle in the tunica media increases.
   a. **Elastic artery**: Elastic arteries function primarily as **conduction arteries**; that is, they conduct blood from the heart to the muscular arteries. Elastic arteries are distinguished by a tunica media with a prominent elastic fiber component that consists of concentric layers of **fenestrated elastic lamellae** (or sheets).

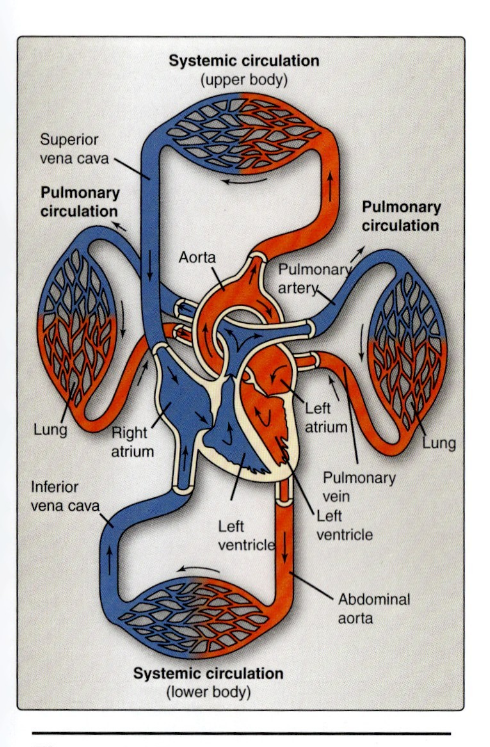

Figure 1.17
Pulmonary and systemic circulations. Red is oxygenated blood; blue is deoxygenated blood.

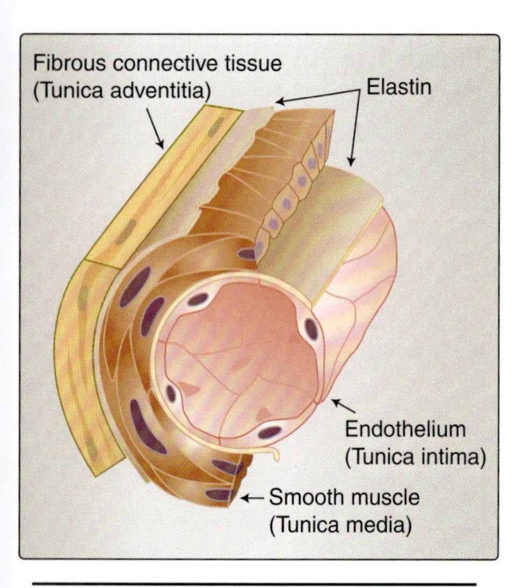

Figure 1.18
Blood vessel structure.

They receive blood under high systolic pressure from the heart and keep the blood circulating while the heart pumps intermittently. Elastic arteries distend during systole and recoil during diastole. Examples include the **pulmonary trunk**, **aorta**, **common carotid arteries**, **subclavian arteries**, and **common iliac arteries**.

b. **Muscular artery**: Muscular arteries function primarily as **distribution arteries**. They have a tunica media with a prominent smooth muscle component that controls the distribution of blood to organs and tissues of the body. Examples include the **axillary**, **ulnar**, **radial**, and **femoral arteries**.

c. **Arteriole**: Arterioles function primarily as **resistance vessels**. They regulate blood flow to the capillary beds. The contraction of the one or two layers of smooth muscle cells in the tunica media increases the vascular resistance and thereby reduces blood flow to the capillary bed. The arterioles offer the greatest resistance to the flow of blood from the heart to the peripheral tissues and therefore play a role in the regulation of **arterial blood pressure**.

d. **Metarteriole**: A metarteriole is the terminal branch of the arterial system and flows directly into the capillary bed. It has a thickened smooth muscle cell layer that acts as a **precapillary sphincter**, regulating blood flow to the capillary bed.

2. **Capillaries**: The vascular wall of a capillary consists of an **endothelium**, a **basal lamina**, and **pericytes**. A pericyte is a cell that has contractile properties and can proliferate in response to tissue injury to act as a stem cell during angiogenesis. The capillary forms a small tube with a diameter that allows for the passage of red blood cells one at a time. Capillaries function primarily as **exchange vessels**. The capillary is the principle site of exchange of water, oxygen, carbon dioxide, glucose, amino acids, proteins, metabolites, and waste products between the blood and cells.

a. **Continuous capillary**: A continuous capillary consists of a single layer of endothelial cells joined by a **zonula occludens** (**tight junction**). It is surrounded by a continuous basal lamina and is found in the lung, muscle, thymus (blood–thymus barrier), nervous system (blood–brain barrier), connective tissue, and exocrine glands.

b. **Fenestrated capillary**: As shown in Figure 1.19, a fenestrated capillary consists of a single layer of endothelial cells joined by a **fascia occludens** (a tight junction that extends only partially around the perimeter of the cell creating small slit-like intercellular spaces). It is surrounded by a continuous basal lamina and has numerous **fenestrae** (or **pores**). The fenestrae are generally bridged by a **diaphragm**. They are found in the kidney (except that in the kidney glomerulus the fenestrated capillary has no diaphragms), lamina propria of the intestine, choroid plexus of the brain, choriocapillaris of the eye, and endocrine glands.

c. **Discontinuous capillary (sinusoid)**: A discontinuous capillary consists of a single layer of endothelial cells joined by a **fascia occludens**. Like fenestrated capillaries, it has numerous **fenestrae**, but its basal lamina is discontinuous. They are found in the liver, bone marrow, and spleen.

and the shoes were a bit large, but they were nonetheless a very comfortable upgrade.

When they got to the emergency room of Nanyuki General Hospital, Dr. Muiruri—Wangai's friend—was there to meet them. After evaluating Jude and running blood tests and X-rays, he determined that Jude was in surprisingly good condition for the ordeal he had been through and only needed a tetanus shot. He advised him to drink plenty of fluids when he got home because his bloodwork indicated that he was still a bit dehydrated.

At the police station, things got more complicated. When they arrived, Wangai's friend—the OCPD—still had not responded to his text message, so they went ahead and presented themselves to the officer at the reception desk and explained the nature of their business. The officer was polite, though unsmiling, and he started jotting down some cursory information in the occurrence book as Jude spoke.

Then, all of a sudden, he stopped writing, and the pen dropped from his hand. An ominous look came over his face. "Stay right where you are, and put your hands up in the air," he said abruptly, rising from his seat and pulling his gun out of his holster. He said something into his walkie-talkie, and three other officers appeared within seconds, their weapons drawn.

"What . . . what's going on?" asked Jude, bewildered, as he turned to Wangai.

Wangai seemed flummoxed as well and had his hands up in the air.

"This is the one we're looking for, sir. You can put your hands down," said one of the officers to Wangai as they patted Jude down and placed him in handcuffs, then began to lead him toward a door that opened into another part of the station.

"Where is Mr. Ochieng, the OCPD?" Wangai asked, somewhat timidly. "I would like to speak to him."

"Ochieng is no longer at this station—he was transferred to Malindi last week. We have a new OCPD—Mr. Shiundu—and I'm getting ready to call him now," replied the officer they had initially spoken to. "Your friend here is a wanted man."

Jude was led into a short hallway with cells on both sides. Through the bars, he could see a few people locked up in twos or threes, seated quietly on the floor in the dim recesses of the cells. When they got to the last one, at the end of the hallway, an officer slid the door open, and Jude was instructed to get inside, after which the door was locked behind him. He was the only occupant of the cell.

"What's going on?" he asked nervously. "Am I under arrest? What did I do?"

"We're just following instructions, sir. You will receive more information when the OCPD gets here," answered one of them as they walked off.

"When . . . when is he coming?"

"Hopefully soon," the same officer called out, after which the door to the hallway slammed shut. Then there was silence and total darkness.

Jude was still sitting in stunned bewilderment when two officers returned half an hour later and brought him out to an interrogation room, where a man who identified himself as Mr. Shiundu—the OCPD—was seated at a table. He was a hefty individual with large, bushy eyebrows and a saturnine disposition. He gestured to Jude to have a seat.

"You're wondering why you're here," he said without any inflection in his voice, so Jude was unsure whether it was a statement or a question. His voice was deep and thundering, with an unmistakable harsh edge to it.

"Yes."

"There are some people who have been very interested in your whereabouts, and they will be coming in tomorrow from Nairobi to talk to you."

"What . . . what people?" Jude asked, his voice faltering.

"You'll find out when they get here."

Jude sighed anxiously, and he could feel his heart pounding in his chest.

"Um . . . sir, I'm an American citizen, and I'd like the embassy notified that I'm here."

The dark eyes studied him menacingly for a few minutes before Shiundu replied, "They know you're here."

"But, Mr. . . . er . . ."

"Shiundu."

"Yes—I'd like to know why I've been arrested."

"You're not under arrest."

"Oh, I'm not? That's good to know," said Jude. "Then can I leave and come back and talk to them tomorrow?"

"Not really."

Jude frowned. "Sir, if I'm not under arrest, then I'd like to leave. And if I'm under arrest, then at least tell me why I've been arrested."

Shiundu leaned forward, and his eyes locked on Jude. "Listen, Mr. Wilson, if that's indeed your name. You're a suspect in a major plot that was just uncovered, and investigators from the antiterrorism force would like to have a word with you, so they will be here to talk to you tomorrow. An alert was issued yesterday to all police stations nationwide to be on the lookout for a number of persons of interest, you being one of them."

"What?" exclaimed Jude incredulously. "Are you kidding me?"

"Young man," replied Shiundu fiercely, "you think this is a game?"

"No, but I think it's pretty far-fetched to accuse me of being involved in terrorist activities. Based on what?"

Shiundu shifted in his seat and let out a loud sigh that sounded like the snorting of an angry bull. His voice got a bit louder.

"Is there anything else I can do for you before tomorrow?"

"Can I get a lawyer?"

"What for?" he asked, seeming genuinely surprised.

"Well, because I'm under arrest for something I didn't do, and I want to make sure—"

"You're not under arrest."

"Oh yeah, I forgot about that. So can I leave now?"

"All right, there doesn't seem to be anything more to talk about," Shiundu said irritably as he rose from his seat. He was burly and stood about six and a half feet tall, so he towered menacingly over Jude, who was still seated. "Is there anything else you would like before I ask my officers to take you back to your cell?"

"Um . . . could I speak to my friend, Wangai—the one I was with earlier this evening?"

Without answering, Shiundu exited the room, so Jude concluded that his request had been denied. He was therefore surprised when he heard the door opening a few minutes later and Wangai being ushered in. Wangai had a meek, confused expression.

"What's going on, my friend?" he asked as the door was shut behind him. "Are you in some sort of trouble?"

"Evidently," said Jude, holding up his handcuffed wrists. "The only thing, though, is that I have no idea what I'm accused of doing. The guy who was here a short while ago said that there was something connected with a terror plot. I have no idea what he's talking about. He said there's people coming in from Nairobi to talk to me, and the American embassy is already aware. I'm not sure I believe him. Also, he told me I'm not under arrest, even though I have these on"—he held up the handcuffs again—"and I can't leave."

Wangai shook his head.

"Is there someone you'd like me to call on your behalf?"

"Please call my mother. I know it's an international call, so I'll make sure I repay any expenses you incur once I get out of here. And also, would you mind calling the American embassy tomorrow morning to make sure they're aware that I'm here?"

"Certainly, don't worry about it," said Wangai eagerly. "Give me your mother's number, and I will call her as soon as I get home. I will call the embassy as well, in the morning."

Then the door opened, and two of Shiundu's underlings appeared.

"Time to go back to your cell, Mr. Wilson," one of them announced.

His eyes briefly met Wangai's; Wangai gave him a reassuring nod, indicating that he would be following up immediately on the tasks that they had discussed.

♒

The next morning, Jude was ushered back into the interrogation room. In the seat Shiundu had been sitting in was a man with a close-cropped hairstyle and an athletic build. He was slouched in his chair, serenely doodling on the blank page of a writing pad that he had on the table in front of him. As Jude lowered himself into the seat, the man looked up and smiled, then nodded to the policeman accompanying Jude, who nodded back and exited the room, leaving them alone.

"Hi, name's Harrison. How are you today?"

Jude stared at him and did not reply.

"I'm guessing you're wondering who I am and why they detained you here."

Silence.

"OK, I guess you do have a right to be ticked off, having spent the night here—I can't imagine the accommodations were any good, with worn-out blankets, paper-thin mattress, and the cold Nanyuki night air tunneling through those slots they have in the wall for ventilation in lieu of windows . . . and, oh gosh, the roaches and bedbugs. It's hard to get any sleep when they're crawling over you. Police cells are tough in this part of the world, I tell you."

Jude had already determined by this point that he didn't like Harrison, who had an unquestionably American accent with a faint trace of a Southern lilt to it.

"I'd like to have a lawyer present," said Jude abruptly.

Harrison smiled and leaned back in his chair. "Do you have one you'd like me to call?"

"Er . . . no, I don't, but I'd like to have one."

Harrison smirked and shrugged his shoulders. "It doesn't work like that over here, Mr. Wilson. See, I just have a few questions that I need answered in a somewhat time-sensitive manner, so I'd really appreciate your cooperation. You're not under arrest—"

Jude snorted and let out a dry laugh. "What is it with you guys? Why do you keep saying I'm not under arrest? I spent the night in a wretched police cell, and I still have handcuffs on. And oh . . . it's not just bedbugs and roaches—did you know about the rats? So I'm not under arrest? What's my status then? Because I wanna get out of here and get on with what's left of my vacation."

"OK, Mr. Wilson, understood. I'll make it quick. What's the purpose of your visit to Kenya?"

"I came to visit the tombs of Lord Baden-Powell and Captain Tom Wilson. And in case you've never heard of them—since it seems that most people haven't—Baden-Powell's an old white dude who founded the Boy Scout movement. Wilson was a scout too. And why would someone like me be interested in them? Because the Boy Scout thing was huge in my family—it's difficult for someone else to understand, but just take it for what it is."

"Got it. Where are they buried?"

"Nyeri."

"All right, are you familiar with a certain Qadir Mohamed—a manager at the YMCA youth hostel in Nairobi?"

"Yeah, very nice guy. He gave me lots of information for my trip to Nyeri, and, from what I hear, many guests go to him for travel tips. I'm here on a budget, so I'm looking to get the most bang for my buck, and he was very helpful in that regard."

"So how did you end up in Nanyuki? This is certainly not the most direct route to Nyeri and, therefore, not the cheapest."

Jude exhaled and shook his head as he began to recount his misadventure involving the taxi.

"What a disaster!" Harrison exclaimed sympathetically when Jude had finished narrating his account. "Even by Nairobi standards, that was a rough ride. So I have a couple more questions. Have you ever sought to join a terrorist group? And number two—do you, or anyone you know, have any links with an organization called Al Shabaab?"

Jude shook his head. "The answer to the first question is no. And I've never even heard of that organization you mentioned."

"OK," said Harrison with a satisfied nod, "that's all the questions I had. Do you have any questions for me? I can't promise I'll answer them, but I'll allow you to ask."

Jude paused for a moment, then proceeded. "Is Harrison your first or last name?"

"Doesn't matter," Harrison replied, his expression taciturn.

"And you're American, right?"

"Maybe—doesn't matter."

"OK. This one matters to me, so I need an answer. Why am I under suspicion of being involved with a terrorist group?"

"Er . . . we have intelligence about some young people coming into this country from the US who are involved in an Al Shabaab plot that was uncovered. We're just trying to make sure we don't let that happen. You suddenly dropped off the radar in Nairobi, and there was concern that you were headed for Isiolo, about an hour from here, which is a major transit point for people heading up into the northeastern part of the country and on to Somalia."

"Oh, I see. But how did anyone know that I had disappeared? Was I being followed?"

A wry smile appeared on Harrison's lips, then he shrugged. "Who knows? We do know that your mother was monitoring the geographic coordinates on your cell phone. I believe you had spoken to her the night before your trip and told her you were traveling to Nyeri the next morning. She looked up your location at around the time you had said you expected to be in Nyeri and was surprised to see the signal indicating that you were headed north toward Nanyuki, instead of to Nyeri. She immediately got concerned, saying that you were not the type of person to change plans on the spur of the moment and certainly not on the way to the destination you'd been wanting to get to for a long time. After trying to call you multiple times without getting a response, the blue dot she was tracking on her screen disappeared, indicating that the phone had likely been turned off. That was the point at which she suspected you were in trouble, and she called the embassy in Nairobi and told them you were missing. It just so happened that this occurred at a time when we have had Westerners landing in Kenya and making their way by land to Somalia with the intention of joining Al Shabaab, which was a possibility that we could not ignore."

Jude shook his head incredulously.

"Any other questions for me?" asked Harrison, getting up to leave.

"Am I free to go now?"

"Yes, sir, you're as free as a bird. I'll have one of the guys come in and take off those bracelets. Sorry you had to spend the night at the station, but I hope you understand what the concern was. I drove in as early as I could from Nairobi so I could try to resolve the issue. And . . . er . . . the guy who found you in the woods—Mr. Wangai—he's out there waiting for you. I interviewed him earlier, and your stories checked out. I hope the rest of your vacation goes well, or at least appreciably better than it has so far."

And with that, Harrison rose and walked out of the room, leaving Jude in quiet contemplation as he waited for an officer to take off his handcuffs and escort him out.

Chapter Eighteen

Wangai lived in an elegant brick house with a well-tended lawn and a dense, carefully manicured spruce hedge on the perimeter. Colorful shrubs and flowers grew in neat array, and there was a man—presumably the gardener—working intently on the beds, pulling out weeds and trimming the bushes. He raised his hand in greeting as Jude and Wangai got out of the car, and Wangai nodded and said something to him in a language Jude didn't understand.

"So this is my home—you didn't get to see much last night when we stopped here before going to the hospital."

"It's beautiful," Jude marveled.

The front door opened, and a girl and boy appeared.

"Hi, Dad!" the girl called out.

"Hi, Wairimu. This is Mr. Wilson—the man I was telling you about this morning. He's from America. Jude, these are my children—Wairimu, who's twelve, and Kioi, who's six."

"Hello, Mr. Wilson," they chimed in unison.

"Oh, you can call me Jude."

They looked at their dad to see if it was OK as, evidently, addressing an adult by their first name was not typical here. Even though he assented, they seemed uncomfortable with it and continued to address him as Mr. Wilson.

Wairimu was the more outgoing child, and she started asking him questions right away, even before he had entered the house. How long was he visiting? Which part of America was he from? Had he ever been to New York?

"Now, now, Wairimu, let's let Mr. Wilson get settled in, then you can ask him all the questions you want to ask. Is that all right?"

"OK," she said, smiling.

After two days in the wilderness and a night in a bug-and-rodent-infested police cell, Jude's first order of business was a shower and change of clothing. There were neat piles of clothes arranged on the dresser for him and fresh plush towels waiting for him in the adjoining bathroom. The hot shower did wonders for his sense of well-being.

When he emerged from the room an hour later, he felt energized and refreshed. He found Wairimu and Kioi sitting quietly in the living room, waiting for him. There was a woman working in the kitchen whose name, Jude learned, was Nkatha. She was petite, in her sixties, and she shuttled quietly between the kitchen and the dining room. A delicious aroma of roast lamb with rosemary seasoning wafted into the living room, and Jude's mouth watered.

"Our dad just went to the shop—he said he'd be back in a few minutes," Wairimu announced.

"OK," said Jude as he plonked himself down in an armchair.

Almost as if by magic, Nkatha appeared, holding a cup of steaming-hot tea, which she set down next to him. She said something to him that he didn't understand, and he smiled and nodded. She had kind, grandmotherly eyes.

"Nkatha said that she would like you to feel welcome and that lunch is almost ready," Wairimu chimed in helpfully.

"Oh, tell her I said thank you."

"She understands English—she just doesn't speak it very well," said Wairimu as Nkatha smiled and returned to the kitchen.

As Wairimu spoke, Kioi sat a short distance away, building something with Lego blocks, glancing shyly in Jude's direction at intervals.

"Do you speak any Kiswahili?" she asked.

"No," replied Jude with a chuckle, shaking his head. "Maybe just a few simple phrases that I learned in my traveler's handbook. Certainly not enough to carry on a conversation, and everyone speaks so fast that I probably wouldn't recognize any of the phrases I learned if someone said them to me."

"Fortunately for you, most people understand some English, so at least they'll understand what you're saying."

"Yeah, that definitely helps."

"Our dad," continued Wairimu, suppressing an awkward smile, "said that you were robbed after getting onto a *haramu* taxi."

"What's that?"

"It's a taxi but not really a taxi. Sometimes bad people will pretend their car is a taxi, then when you get in, they take you somewhere and rob you."

"Oh yeah—that was a big mess. They took everything—my wallet, my passport—everything. A lady who got into the vehicle—I thought she was a passenger sharing my ride—gave me something to eat, and I fell asleep. When I regained consciousness, I was out in the bush all by myself. They took my shoes, my belt, jacket . . . everything. . . . I'm really glad your dad found me when he did because it was getting dark, and apparently there were some hyenas trailing me."

"I'm sure the hyenas weren't very happy that dinner got canceled," Wairimu said, smiling wryly.

"Yup, I don't think they were laughing anymore when I got into your dad's car."

Kioi evidently found the statements about the hyenas and their dinner very amusing, and he giggled bashfully before softly echoing, "Too bad for the hyenas."

Jude turned to him and grinned. "That's right, Kioi—too bad for them. So what grade are you guys in?"

"Standard one," replied Kioi in a barely audible voice.

"And how about you, Wairimu?"

"I'm in standard six."

"Hmm . . . from your ages, I'm gonna guess that standard one and standard six are like first grade and sixth grade in America."

Wairimu shrugged and shook her head to indicate that she had no idea if that was indeed the case. Just then, there was the jiggling of a key in the front door, and Wangai entered the house with two large bags of groceries, which he ferried into the kitchen before coming back to where Jude and the kids were sitting.

"Feeling better after a shower and a cup of tea?"

"Absolutely!"

"Excellent. Lunch is almost ready, after which we can show you the farm. That way, you can enjoy some fresh air, and these youngsters can get a bit of exercise. Right, kids?"

Wairimu and Kioi nodded dutifully, though the mention of a walk through the farm didn't appear to evoke the same level of enthusiasm in them that it did in their father.

"And before I forget, Jude, your mother asked me to call her this morning with an update, so we should call her after lunch. She'll be very excited to speak to you and to learn that the whole situation with the cops got resolved. I didn't manage to call the embassy because the police told me I had to be back at the station before seven, to give my account of how I met you and all the events leading up to when we reported to the station."

Wangai turned his attention toward the dining room as Nkatha started bringing steaming dishes from the kitchen and placing them on the dinner table. In a soft voice, she said something to Wangai in Kiswahili. "Thank you, Nkatha," he said before turning to Jude. "Lunch is ready. Nkatha makes the best lamb on this side of Mount Kenya, and it's most delicious while it's still hot, so let's get to the table before it starts to get cold."

As they calmly sauntered through Wangai's bucolic ten-acre farm that afternoon—where he kept about fifty dairy cows and grew maize and an array of different vegetables—Jude was mellow and relaxed. Wangai and his family were very likable, and even Jude's mother seemed to have formed a connection with Wangai, chatting with him for a good ten minutes after she was done talking to Jude. And she did indicate that Scoutmaster Wilson, who was sitting by her side as she spoke, had a big smile on his face and gave a hearty thumbs-up with his left hand. Jude had decided that he didn't want his parents to worry more than they already had, so he felt it best not to tell them the reason Mr. Harrison had given for his being in police custody, stating simply that it was a case of mistaken identity.

They got past the large barns where the cows were housed. The ground inclined steeply from there, all the way to a hedge that demarcated the end of Wangai's land and the beginning of the neighboring property.

"I think we should turn around here," said Wangai. "Going down the slope is one thing, but coming back up carrying this young fellow here"—he pointed to Kioi—"is a bit of a challenge. Take my word for it—I've had to do it a few times, and he's only gotten bigger since."

As they turned around, Wairimu asked, "Dad, can we show him where Mom is buried?"

Wangai hesitated momentarily, then shrugged. "OK, Wairimu—you lead the way."

As they walked, Jude pondered what he had just heard. He had noticed a beautiful, smiling young woman in a number of the photographs in the living room, but there had been no mention of any other member of the household besides the people he'd already met. When they passed through the small gate that separated the farm from the house and immediate environs, Wairimu headed toward a weeping willow tree that was close to the perimeter of the property. There, at the foot of the tree, was an ornate marble gravestone that read:

Anne Njeri Wangai
Born: March 5th 1973
Died: August 19th 2016
“We will see you again.”

A subdued silence fell over them, and Jude respectfully directed his gaze downward. It was Wairimu who spoke first.

“My mother died of breast cancer two years ago,” she stated in a matter-of-fact tone.

“I’m very sorry to hear that,” Jude replied.

Wangai didn’t speak. It was only when they turned around and started heading back to the house that he said, reflectively, his voice quivering with emotion, “Anne was a special person—one can never fully recover from losing someone like that. Had it not been for the fact that Nkatha was living with us—helping take care of the kids and keep the household going—I’d have lost my mind. That was a tough year.”

“Nkatha,” Wairimu volunteered, “is like a grandma to Kioi and me. She was living with our parents even before Kioi and I were born.”

"Hmm . . . yes, that's right—I think she moved in with us in 1999, if I remember correctly," mused Wangai. "Anne and I had been married for about a year when Nkatha moved in with us. But we knew her even before that because we used to buy fruits from her stall at the market. That's how we met her. She used to sell these gorgeous mangoes, which are normally very hard to find, from a place called Tharaka. She's originally from there. My wife could never get enough of those mangoes, so we made the slightest excuse to go to the market whenever mangoes were in season.

"Then, one day, some rich fella started eyeing the plot of land where the open-air market was—the next thing we knew, the sellers at the market were given twenty-four hours to vacate their lots. Many of them protested, but when armed policemen showed up at six o'clock the next morning, paving the way for the bulldozers, the people at the market knew they didn't stand a chance. As soon as we heard about it, my wife called Nkatha on her mobile phone. In her last year at the market, whenever she got a shipment of mangoes, she would send my wife a text message to let her know that she had set aside a juicy batch for her.

"The day of the demolition, when Anne called Nkatha, she was weighing her limited options. She was contemplating going back to Tharaka, although there was really nothing to go back to—she'd been married before, but her husband divorced her because they were unable to have children, which he considered her fault. All her in-laws shunned her as well. Her family was poor, and they also rejected her for having 'failed her husband' and for having been divorced, so she took her meager belongings and came out here to start a new life for herself in Nanyuki. Anne offered her a job as a housekeeper and invited her to live with us. That, in hindsight, was one of the best things that happened to us. Sometimes you get rewarded in life for helping people in ways that may not seem like a big deal to you. Who knew that the person we were 'saving' back then would turn out to be the person that would hold everything together in this household during the two years that Anne battled cancer and in the time that has elapsed since she passed away?"

Jude nodded silently, unsure of what to say, as they walked up the steps to the front door of the house.

"Life comes with its share of pain, but there's often sweetness hidden inside—it's often difficult to appreciate the sweetness until after the pain has passed," reflected Wangai as he opened the door to the house.

Chapter Nineteen

After all the drama associated with his trip, Jude had pretty much given up trying to get to Nyeri and was planning on getting back to Nairobi and making a beeline for the American embassy in order to process temporary travel documents for his flight home. He had no money, which meant that he hadn't yet figured out how he would pay for the cost of travel back to Nairobi, as well as meals for the week or so before his flight and even the taxi to the airport. On the day he was released from police custody, he'd called his bank and credit card company—a hugely complex undertaking in itself—and reported his cards stolen, at which point, they were immediately deactivated. So here he was in a foreign country with no passport, credit card, or money . . .

He was mortified by the idea of asking Wangai for money. It seemed rather crude and presumptuous to do so. On the other hand, he was the person who had watched the entire situation unfold, so not much of an explanation was needed. His other alternative was to have his mother wire him some money. The only problem with that, though, was that he would need identification documents in order to claim the money, and in order to travel to the embassy to get identification documents, he needed money. He was quietly ruminating over this quandary on the evening of the second day, when Wangai asked, “When were you thinking of going to visit Baden-Powell’s grave?”

Jude was startled for a moment because he didn’t remember having mentioned this to his host.

“Isn’t that where you told me you had been traveling to when you left Nairobi? I remember you mentioning that when I picked you up in the bush.”

“Oh yeah! Well . . . um . . . I don’t really think that’s an option for me now. I just need to figure out how to get to Nairobi so I can get my emergency travel documents in time for my flight at the end of next week.”

“You must be joking,” exclaimed Wangai as he erupted with incredulous laughter. “You came *all this way*, and now you’re going to turn around and go back when you’re just one hour away from your destination? No, no, no . . . that’s not how we’re going to do this.”

“Well, I don’t have a single penny in my pocket, so there’s not exactly a choice to be made.”

“Don’t worry about the money, my friend. I can take you to Nyeri and then Nairobi in one day. We can do it this Saturday, if you like. Even if we make a leisurely trip, I’ll have you at the YMCA youth hostel by four o’clock.”

Jude was immediately filled with a mixture of gratitude and embarrassment. “Oh, that’d be too much to expect you to not only take me to Nairobi, but to go through Nyeri as well. If I remember from the map, Nyeri is in the other direction.”

Wangai laughed heartily, a bright twinkle in his eyes. “I see that you’re one of those people who feel they have to be able to reciprocate any kindness they’re about to receive. But what if you have nothing to give yet still need help? Then what? Look at it this way—if I showed up outside your house in Seattle, with no money, no shoes, and no passport and needed help, would you help me get to where I needed to go? If so, then I’m just doing for you what you would do for me. And even if you wouldn’t necessarily consider helping me in that situation, it still doesn’t leave you with any options for getting back to Nairobi here and now. Unless, of course, you want to take the Samosa Express again? That didn’t work out so well the first time, did it?”

“No, it didn’t,” said Jude, grinning. “It didn’t work out very well.”

“OK, let’s plan on going Saturday morning. I grew up in Nyeri, so I know exactly where Baden-Powell’s tomb is. I went to Saint Peter’s church as a kid—I think it’s a cathedral now—which is where the cemetery is, and I always wondered why foreigners came to visit that gravesite. Little did I know that one day I'd be driving one such person there, many years later."

≈

On the day before they left Nanyuki, Jude got to stand on the equator, which passed through the town. Besides a somewhat weather-beaten yellow-and-black signpost marking the famed location, there wasn't much else. He posed triumphantly next to the sign, with Wairimu and Kioi on either side of him, as Wangai snapped photos on his cell phone.

That evening, Nkatha surprised him with a sumptuous dinner of baked rainbow trout with *pilau* (flavored rice) and a delectable assortment of grilled vegetables from Wangai's farm. Evidently, the choice of trout had been influenced by a conversation two days prior, in which Jude—in response to a question from Kioi regarding his favorite food—had waxed eloquent about his mother's amazing salmon and trout recipes. During the discussion, which took place on a quiet, lazy afternoon, Nkatha stopped in a couple of times—once to clear the remaining dishes from the lunch table and then to bring him a steaming cup of tea—and she had not appeared to be listening to the conversation. It was, therefore, quite surprising when, on the eve of his departure, she served the dinner and said proudly to him, in broken English, "Today, you eat fish, just like at your home—because even here is your home!"

She was beaming widely when she said it, and the astonished responses from Wangai and his children indicated that this meal was not part of her usual repertoire.

"Nkatha, I didn't even know that you cooked fish. The trout is delicious," exclaimed Wangai.

"Thank you, Nkatha," said Jude, a wide grin on his face.

She nodded courteously and returned to the kitchen.

After that, Jude started to experience conflicting emotions about his departure from the Wangai residence. On one hand, he was excited about going to Nyeri and accomplishing the primary purpose of his visit. On the other hand, however, his days at Wangai's home had been so blissful and relaxing that his day of departure seemed to have come too soon.

Early the next morning, as the rays of the sun began to thaw out the frosty ground, Jude, Wangai, and the children climbed into the car, waved goodbye to Nkatha, and began their journey to Nyeri. Mount Kenya was not visible from Wangai's home, but as soon as they got onto the highway, they could see it in its imposing grandeur, basking in the golden rays of the rising sun. Jude feverishly snapped photos of it on Wangai's phone, hoping to capture the magic of the moment to show his parents when he got home. Wangai had promised to email him the pictures.

"You can never see enough of that mountain," Wangai said. "I still marvel at it despite having lived in the area around it for most of my life."

Jude nodded in agreement.

It took them about an hour to get to Nyeri. The children had fallen asleep as soon as the car tires made contact with the asphalt on the highway, and a rhythmic sound of soft snoring emanated from the back seat. Since it was an early Saturday morning, there weren't many cars or pedestrians in the streets, so Wangai drove slowly and leisurely, pointing out interesting sights along the way.

"See that big colorful sign on that three-story building over there, the one that reads 'Nyam's Jams'?

"I went to primary school with the owner of that building—a very successful businesswoman called Nyambura, who owns numerous properties in town. That particular one is probably the trendiest nightspot within a radius of maybe a hundred kilometers. Young people come all the way from Nanyuki just so they can say they went to Nyam's Jams. Nyambura used to sell stuff all the time, even in lower primary school. She'd bring random things, like colored pencils, marbles, and plastic bangles, and exchange them for things she wanted, such as felt pens, notebooks, stickers, cookies—you name it—usually getting pretty good deals from her less savvy classmates.

"When I heard about the new nightclub, I was very amused because the name was quite ironic; I remembered one of her childhood ventures when she tried to make plum jam and sell it. It didn't go so well because she'd basically mashed up the plums and added sugar, so the final product wasn't very tasty. But the thing about her is that if one project failed, she didn't beat herself up about it. She just moved on to the next thing. I see her every now and then when I'm in Nyeri. She's quite a lively and down-to-earth person—very fun to be around—and every time I talk to her, she'll tell me about the next great business ideas she's thought of, some of which have succeeded marvelously over the years.

"You see that shop over there?" said Wangai, pointing out a grocery store as they slowed down at an intersection.

"Yeah?"

"That's the oldest shop in Nyeri—it's been around since the early 1900s. During the colonial days, it had a sign outside that said 'Dogs and Africans Not Allowed.'"

Jude cringed.

"Yes, that's our history. Now it caters mainly to Africans," Wangai continued. "The dogs are still waiting their turn." With that last statement, he roared with merry laughter until tears started streaming down his face.

In the back seat, the children stirred awake from the noise, and Kioi asked, in a drowsy voice, "Are we there yet?"

"Yes, Kioi, we have just arrived in Nyeri."

"Yay! Can we buy mandazi?"

"We'll see about that, young man; we will see," said Wangai with a wide grin. There was excited whispering in the back seat because, apparently, that expression was known to be as good as a yes.

Wairimu spoke next. "So, Mr. Wilson, I still don't understand why you came all this way to see the graves of people who aren't even related to you."

Jude smiled. "Yes, Wairimu—it does seem a bit strange, doesn't it? Well, when I was your age, I used to be a scout, and my father was the scoutmaster, the adult in charge. Daddy loved everything about scouting, and he and I ended up doing lots of things together, like camping in the woods, practicing how to tie different types of knots . . . things like that. When he was a young man, he met Captain Wilson, who was a scoutmaster, and because they had the same exact name, my dad felt drawn to scouting. When we learned that Captain Wilson was buried in the same graveyard as Lord Baden-Powell, we talked about how it would be a great idea to visit that cemetery."

"Did your dad want to come as well?"

"If there was one place he could visit in the world, Wairimu, this would have been it. But he's not much of a traveler, so he was quite happy to visit it in his imagination only. Besides, he had a stroke a few months ago, so even if he'd wanted to come, it would have been very difficult for him to travel. So I'm doing this for him and for me . . ."

Jude swallowed hard, and a brief pause followed.

"What's a stroke?" Kioi piped up.

"Oh, it's when a part of your brain doesn't get enough blood, so it quits working, then you're not able to move your arms or legs or, sometimes, talk. My dad can't move his right hand anymore, and he's not able to talk, although he understands when you talk to him."

"What makes part of the brain not get enough blood while the other parts do?" pursued Kioi, seemingly fascinated.

"Kioi, let me explain it to you because I learnt it in school the other day," said Wairimu authoritatively. "Remember, when I showed you how to put your finger on your wrist to check your pulse, and there was something throbbing under your skin? That's an artery, and they're the ones that take blood everywhere. So if one of the arteries going into your brain gets blocked, then the blood can't reach your brain, and the cells in that part of your brain die."

"What's a cell?" Kioi asked innocently.

Wairimu let out a big sigh. "Don't worry, little brother—when you're as big as me, it will all make sense," she declared reassuringly.

Jude and Wangai listened in quiet amusement.

They arrived at their destination, a white-walled cottage with black trim and a brick-red corrugated iron roof, nestled in a picturesque grove of trees, with a well-kept lawn and carefully trimmed hedges and bushes. Wangai brought the car to a stop in front of the building, and they got out. There was a faded wooden sign that read:

PAXTU

HOME OF THE FOUNDER OF THE WORLDWIDE BOY SCOUT AND GIRL GUIDE MOVEMENTS LORD ROBERT BADEN POWELL OM, GCMG, GCVO, KCB, BARON OF GILWELL. ALSO REMEMBERED AS "HERO OF THE SEIGE [SIC] OF MAFEKING" DURING THE GREAT BOER WAR IN SOUTH AFRICA 1891–1900.

THIS COTTAGE WAS LATER OCCUPIED BY

JIM CORBETT

DESTROYER OF THE MAN EATING TIGERS IN CENTRAL INDIA DURING THE 1920–30C. THE ADJACENT MUSEUM IS DEDICATED TO THE SCOUTING TRADITIONS OF THE WORLD.

ENTRANCE FEE KSHS 300 PER PERSON

FREE TO UNIFORMED SCOUTS AND GUIDES

Wangai slowly shook his head as he read aloud the words, then let out a low whistle. "'Look at all those letters behind Baden-Powell's name. I'd be interested to know what the people of Mafeking think of him since it's unlikely he was a hero to both sides in that siege."

Jude smiled and shrugged.

"As for the 'Destroyer of the Man-eating Tigers' . . . he should have insisted they add the initials DMETCI after his name, so he could keep up with the first guy," Wangai continued with a chuckle. "Even without knowing what the letters behind Baden-Powell's name stand for, it seems to me that this Corbett the tiger slayer is the guy you don't want to mess with."

"Dad, are there really man-eating tigers?" Kioi asked hesitantly as they walked toward the cottage.

"Well, Kioi, I think any tiger that's hungry enough will eat a man. But if Mr. Corbett here is to be believed, the people of central India have nothing to worry about anymore. And neither do you, because the only tigers in Africa are the ones in zoos. Let's go inside and you ask the guides. And after we're done here, we can go and get some mandazi, after which we can take Mr. Wilson to where Baden-Powell and Captain Wilson are buried."

≈

Jude spent over an hour at the cemetery adjacent to Saint Peter's Cathedral. Time went by much quicker than he'd anticipated. After the initial ten minutes or so, during which he stood in numb incredulity, overwhelmed by the fact that he was finally standing by the graves that he'd traveled almost ten thousand miles to see, other emotions began to well up within him—feelings of unassailable triumph at having accomplished his mission, mixed with profound reverence for where he was, as well as deep sadness that his dad couldn't be there to share the moment with him.

In the midst of his reveries, he caught sight of the gardener coming in his direction, trundling a rickety wheelbarrow laden with implements of his trade.

"*Habari?* [How're you doing?]"

"*Mzuri sana* [Very good]," replied Jude, using one of the few Swahili phrases he had mastered thus far in his sojourn.

"You came at a good time," continued the gardener in confident, though accented English, most notable for the way he used the sounds "r" and "l" interchangeably, so that the words "slope" and "broken" might sound more like "srope" and "bloken." "We are expecting a lot of people this afternoon—I think I heard the provost saying there were four tour buses scheduled to come in today."

"Wow," exclaimed Jude.

The gardener introduced himself as Preston Njoroge. He was slender, probably in his mid-to-late forties, with close-cropped hair and a dark scar on his left cheek shaped like an upside-down *Y*. His manner was amiable and easygoing, and he seemed intent on not passing up the opportunity to chat with a living human being.

"When I first saw you, I thought you were a Kenyan, but now that I've heard you speak, I can see that you are not from here."

"No," said Jude with a smile, "I'm an American—just another tourist, like the ones coming this afternoon."

"That's OK. Most of the people that come here are tourists."

As they chatted, Jude learned that Njoroge had been tending the grounds of the cemetery for twenty-two years, a fact of which he was immensely proud.

"When I started working here, I was just a young man, even younger than you. I'd been hoping to move to Nairobi to live with my uncle when this job came up. I thought I'd do it for a few months and save some money while I applied for a job in Nairobi. That was more than twenty years ago. Now, I have a wife and three children, and I'm still here tending to these graves. It's very peaceful, and most of the time, the only thing I'm listening to is my thoughts or singing. I usually finish my work before the visitors get here, then I go over to the main church compound and do my other duties."

"Sounds like you're happy here," observed Jude.

"Very much so. I enjoy the peace and quiet. It doesn't pay very much, but my wife and I run a kiosk downtown, and with our income from here and the kiosk, we're able to get by. So are you a scout, like most of the people that come here?"

"I was when I was younger. My father was a scoutmaster, too, but he wasn't able to make this trip."

"*Pole sana* [I'm sorry to hear that]."

There was a short pause, then Njoroge bent down to pick up the handlebars of his wheelbarrow with the intention of proceeding to where he had been going. Jude cleared his throat hesitantly and said, "Er . . . do you know much about the people buried here?"

Njoroge looked up quizzically. "You mean like what they were like when they were alive?"

"Yeah."

"Not really, though with Baden-Powell, I know from what many visitors say that he is a very respected figure in the Boy Scout movement. They have guides who have a lot more information at Paxtu, his cottage, if you haven't been there."

"I was already there, and I listened to the guide," said Jude, somewhat wearily. "I guess what I'm trying to find out is

. . . er . . . like what do . . . what do locals like you think of the people buried here?"

Njoroge paused in concentration, then shook his head in resignation. "I'm not really sure I understand your question."

Jude sighed. "OK, let me see if I can explain. You already told me that lots of tourists come here. However, when I arrived in the country and took a taxi from the airport, the taxi driver didn't seem to have any idea who I was talking about. It's happened with a few other people. So it just seems rather odd to me that I've come all this way, and the locals don't even seem to know about him, or care, for that matter."

"Oh, I see what you're asking," said Njoroge as he nodded slowly, still with a pensive look on his face. "Hmm . . . I guess, to most Kenyans, these settlers came here to live their own lives, not really caring about the lives of Africans, so they wouldn't be considered heroes. Some of the colonialists were actually terrible people, so there may not be a reason to want to remember them."

"Do you know anything about the guy buried there, at the corner of the cemetery—under that tree?"

Njoroge looked up in the direction Jude was pointing, and an unmistakable frown came over his face.

"Who, Wilson?"

"Yes."

"Nobody comes to see Wilson," he said dismissively before bending over and grabbing the handles of his wheelbarrow.

"Wait . . . is there something I need to know about Wilson? From the way you reacted, he doesn't seem to have been a popular guy around here."

Njoroge let out a heavy sigh, and there was suddenly a hard expression in his eyes. "Wilson is dead, like he should be. My job doesn't pay me very much, but one of the benefits I have is that I get to trample every day on the grave of the dog who killed my grandfather. That Wilson was an animal. He and his men came and arrested several people from my village, including my grandfather, my father, and several of my uncles. Wilson and his men suspected that my grandfather was one of the Mau Mau ringleaders in my community, and they beat him daily and tortured him, but he wouldn't confess. Then, one day, as they were harassing him, standing around him as he was seated on the ground, Wilson suddenly took a hammer and just started bashing my grandfather in the head until his brains leaked out of his skull. That dog there killed my grandfather!"

Njoroge's whole body was quivering with rage that had been suppressed over several years.

"You know what, Mr. . . . er . . . Mr. . . ."

Jude quickly said his first name, deducing that using his last name—Wilson—would have been awkward in this situation.

"Mr. Jude—that's a nice name. You see, Mr. Jude, since you are interested in hearing more than the simple stories they tell the other tourists, I'm going to tell you something that I've never told anyone else, not even my wife," Njoroge continued, bringing his voice down to an urgent but conspiratorial whisper. "Did you manage to get close to Wilson's grave?"

"I did."

"Did you notice anything unusual?"

"Well . . . er . . . the grass is greener in that corner of the graveyard . . ."

"*Ehe* . . . ?" Njoroge urged him on eagerly.

"Yeah, that's about all I noticed. Why?"

"Did you notice an unusual smell?"

Jude hesitated. "Well, it did smell a little damp and funky, but I figured that was because it was in the shade."

Njoroge chuckled gleefully, rubbing his hands with satisfaction.

"Mr. Jude, you know how they wish dead people to rest in peace? Well, for Captain Wilson there, it's a different word than 'peace,' but it sounds similar. I make sure he gets lots of it. In fact, every morning, I'll drink a big cup of chai at home, and I don't stop at any bathroom—I go straight there and deliver my morning greeting to that animal. I know it's not going to bring back my grandfather, but it still feels good to know that the most frequent visitor to Wilson's grave is the person that comes to urinate on it."

Jude was flabbergasted but also rather amused.

"Well, Mr. Jude," said Njoroge, "it was very nice to meet you and I hope you enjoy the rest of your stay in Kenya. And about the . . . er . . . thing with the grave . . ."

"I won't say a word," replied Jude reassuringly, eliciting a grateful smile from Njoroge.

"Have a nice day then."

Jude had turned around and started walking toward the main entrance of the compound, when he saw Wangai approaching.

"I thought I'd come and check if you wanted to take any pictures to show people when you go back home," he said cheerily. "The kids are waiting in the car. Neither of them wants to come into a graveyard."

"Sure, that'd be great."

Jude turned back, and the two walked first to Baden-Powell's grave, then to Captain Wilson's. By the time Wangai arrived, Njoroge had disappeared off somewhere. As they got close to Wilson's grave, and Jude squatted to pose next to the headstone, Wangai crinkled his nose.

"Hmm . . . there's an odd smell around here. I wonder if it's coming from that tree. If we weren't in a graveyard, I'd have assumed it was something else."

"It's probably the tree," said Jude, posing with a wide grin as Wangai clicked on his cell phone and started taking pictures.

Chapter Twenty

The drive back to Nairobi was uneventful, and the only traffic they encountered was in Pangani, on the outskirts of the city. Kioi and Wairimu had fallen asleep the minute the vehicle exited the gates of Saint Peter's Cathedral, and they did not awaken until the car came to a standstill in the parking lot of the YMCA. Along the way, Jude and Wangai conversed intermittently; for the most part, however, each was engaged in his own quiet, meandering rumination.

Jude was surprised to find Qadir in the lobby when he went to the front desk to request a room key, his other one having been lost in the samosa incident.

"Oh, hi, Qadir. I didn't expect to find you here on a Saturday. I thought you only worked weekdays."

Qadir grinned as the two exchanged a hearty handshake.

"I just wanted to make sure you were OK after your ordeal, especially since you lost all your documents and money. And don't worry about your accommodation for the remaining days of your stay—my higher-ups said that it was

OK for you to wire us the balance whenever you're able to, once you get back to the States."

"Oh, thank you. That's very kind of you. Actually, do you have a moment? I'd like you to meet my friends—they're outside in the car. Mr. Wangai is the kind soul who found me wandering in the forest, and I've been staying with him and his family since."

Qadir gladly obliged, and they strode to where Wangai and his children were waiting. An enthusiastic exchange of greetings ensued.

"Mr. Wilson, is this your brother?" Kioi piped up amid the spirited conversation.

Jude and Qadir chortled gleefully.

"No, Kioi, Mr. Qadir is the manager of this place," said Jude. "Why do you ask—do we look alike?"

"A little," replied Kioi timidly, his voice barely above a whisper.

"Well, I've heard that if you get along with someone and you spend time together, you could sometimes start to look alike," Jude said to Kioi with a grin.

Wangai popped open the trunk of his car and retrieved the small bag containing Jude's belongings, primarily toiletries and items of clothing donated by his host. Somewhere along the drive, as they neared Nairobi, he'd slipped Jude an envelope containing 20,000 shillings—about $200—for his upkeep in the remaining days of his stay in Kenya.

"Oh, I really can't," protested Jude weakly when Wangai held out the envelope.

"Don't be ridiculous, my friend. How else do you plan on getting by for the remaining days you have left in the country?"

"Well, thank you. I really appreciate it."

"Don't mention it. Remember what I said before—I'm just doing for you what I believe you'd do for me if I showed up stranded at your doorstep in America."

Now, as they started to say their goodbyes, Jude felt profound feelings of gratitude and sadness as he reflected on the fortuitous way his path had intersected with that of the Wangai family.

"Make sure you come and visit again," said Wairimu, the buoyancy in her voice just barely masking the rising wistfulness she was feeling within.

Tears were already streaming down Kioi's cheeks, and Jude swallowed hard as he tried to maintain his composure. "I'll definitely try to come and visit again, Kioi. And if for some reason I can't, then you'll have to come and visit me in America, right?"

"OK," Kioi said between sniffles, managing a smile as he clambered into the vehicle, and Jude and Qadir stepped back to make way as it slowly began to back out of the parking space.

♒

Jude spent Sunday morning lounging idly on the terrace that overlooked the swimming pool. His flight home was at the end of the week, and after the drama-filled stay he'd had so far, he relished the prospect of an uneventful remainder of his stay. At about ten am, the receptionist had patched through a call from his mother to the landline in his room.

"Mom, how did you think to call the front desk? And where did you even get the number?" he asked incredulously.

"Everything's on the internet nowadays, Jude—it's really not that complicated. Besides, how else was I supposed to call you after Joshua dropped you off? I spoke to him yesterday, and he told me you'd arrived OK. What a fine young man. I enjoyed speaking with him while you were at his house, and I promised to keep in touch with him even in your absence. Dad and I are looking forward to your return at the end of the week."

"I'm looking forward to coming home as well, Mom. It's been a great adventure—it truly has—but I can't wait to get back home."

They spoke for an hour, and after he hung up, he decided to take a stroll to Uhuru Park that afternoon. By around two o'clock, when he set out, all the busy Sunday morning traffic from the cluster of churches at the intersection of State House Road, Nyerere Road, and University Way had abated, giving way to scores of pedestrians meandering casually as they enjoyed the sublime sunny afternoon. Every other moment, a cyclist or two zipped down State House Road, triumphantly celebrating the solitary day of reprieve from the notoriously aggressive Nairobi drivers who tormented them the rest of the week.

At Uhuru Park, families picnicked and lazed around while others drifted in rental paddleboats in the murky green waters of the artificial pond at the center of the park. Right at the corner of the park, next to Kenyatta Avenue, a street preacher roared animatedly into his microphone—his hoarse proclamations amplified by two giant speakers positioned close by—to an enthralled crowd of about fifty, who applauded enthusiastically every now and then.

Kenya was unlike anything he'd imagined it would be, and even with the misadventure he'd had, the trip had still been a glorious experience. His mind drifted to Captain Wilson. It was rather ironic that the thing that had inspired his trip had ended up an ignominious footnote, needing to be delicately circumvented, if possible, when he retold his adventures back home. He'd already decided he would not share any of the derogatory new information with his dad, much of whose life had been inspired by the captain and who now, in poor health after his stroke, could only be harmed by this new discovery. He found himself a spot and, sprawling out on the grass, began to bask sedately like a few other people around him. He was going to miss this place.

Chapter Twenty-One

Jude was a little confused when he first saw the circular arrangement of rocks on the patch of grass, adjacent to the walkway, close to where his favorite table was on the terrace. He glanced around quizzically, but everyone seemed to be minding their own business, so he shrugged and took a seat at the table, waiting for a server to appear. It wasn't long before Ogutu—one of the waiters he'd become familiar with—showed up.

"Good morning, Mr. Wilson, welcome back from your safari. Will it be the usual today?" Ogutu said heartily.

Jude returned the greeting and nodded. He'd had coffee and mandazi for the first couple of days of his stay in Nairobi and had been considering trying out other items on the menu, but he'd liked the feeling of familiarity when a server asked if he wanted the "usual," so he'd said yes. This had become his routine for the week or so before he set out on the eventful trip to Nyeri. When he got back to the YMCA, he was pleased to see that they hadn't forgotten his preferred breakfast.

"Er, Ogutu . . . would you happen to know . . . ?" he began, pointing at the rocks in the grass.

Ogutu chuckled and grinned awkwardly as he started to walk toward the kitchen.

"You'll have to ask Mr. Qadir about that. That was his idea."

Jude was bemused. As he sat back and awaited his breakfast, his eyes went back to the circle of rocks, with a large solitary one in the center. Then he gazed around pensively at the handful of people lounging on the terrace and the few lap swimmers gracefully plying the clear blue water in the pool. He was lost in thought when Qadir's exuberant greeting roused him back to reality.

"Oh, hey, Qadir, how are you today? I didn't see you coming."

"I'm very well. I hope you had a good day yesterday."

"I did. I spent it in Uhuru Park watching other people whiling away their Sunday afternoon. Very relaxing—a nice way to remember my last weekend in the city."

Ogutu arrived with the coffee and mandazi, quietly placing them on the table, then departed.

"Oh, before I forget," continued Jude, "what's with *that*?" He pointed at the circle of rocks in the grass.

An embarrassed grin appeared on Qadir's face. "That was supposed to be put there on Friday—the day of your departure—but I should have known better than to give Njagi, our groundskeeper, any instructions that weren't supposed to take effect immediately. Everything for him is right away, and he often rushes off to begin a task before he's heard all the instructions. See, while you were away, I did a little reading about that scouting movement you belong to, and I saw this sign with a circle with a dot in it, which I guess is a sign meant to signify that someone has gone home. I knew you were leaving on Friday night, so I'd planned to have this placed here that morning at a location where you would see it, since we all know this is the table you come to for breakfast. Unfortunately, my man Njagi ruined the surprise. It wasn't until Ogutu came out to take your order and saw it that we realized it was there. So it's not much of a—" Qadir shifted his eyes to a spot behind Jude and lifted his hand to greet someone there. "Oh, hey, Mr. Momanyi, *habari ya asubuhi.*"[20]

When Jude turned around to see who it was, his heart stopped.

"Good morning, gentlemen. Have a seat."

Qadir looked confused, but the man gestured to a seat, and he himself pulled up a chair and sat down before placing a printout on the table in front of each of them. Jude peered at the document, which had his name and date of birth at the top.

"Go on, you can take it. It's yours. I have some information that you might find useful. You're wondering

[20] Good morning.

where you've seen me before?" He turned to Jude. "Yes, that was me in Nanyuki."

"Mr. Harrison?"

"Maybe—whatever I told you my name was. It doesn't matter. Anyway, here's the information I have, and you may do with it as you please. I'm only going to tell you what you need to know, and no, I will not answer any questions. Some DNA samples were obtained as part of an investigation into an imminent threat involving an unspecified number of individuals who were planning on traveling to Kenya from the US, with a view to making it up north to Somalia to join ranks with Al Shabaab, the terrorist organization. You arrived in the country at the time of the alert. When you took a trip out of Nairobi and dropped off the radar, we got involved—I already explained this to you when we met in Nanyuki. Regarding why I'm here: our lab guy, who's somewhat of a savant in pattern recognition, pulls both your reports from a stack of about seventy and says to me, 'Are these guys related? I know this isn't a sibling DNA test, but there's about a forty-seven percent overlap in their sequences, which is pretty high for two fellas with totally different names from different parts of the world.'

"It might be something. It might be nothing. I'm not a DNA expert, but it's not every day that Aziz, my lab guy, comes to me with strong feelings about a random finding in his mountain of spreadsheets, so I figured I'd pass on the information to you, and you can decide what to do with it. That's all I had, gentlemen. I'm going to walk away now, and let's hope never to meet again."

And with that, the man—Mr. Harrison or Momanyi, whichever it was—pushed back his seat, rose to his feet, and strode off toward the main entrance of the building, leaving Jude and Qadir stunned, poring hesitantly over the jargon-filled transcripts but seemingly even more perplexed at the identity of the mysterious interlocutor.

"That's the guy who interrogated me when I was in police custody in Nanyuki. At the time, I could have sworn he was American, but now, I'm not so sure. He sounds foreign, maybe even British."

Qadir shook his head incredulously. "That's the first time I've ever heard him speak English. He's been coming here regularly the past few months. When we first met, he said he was a businessman from Kitale, a town in western Kenya. The only language I've ever heard him speak is Kiswahili, though his Kiswahili is rather strange—very proper and grammatical, like Tanzanian Kiswahili. Kenyan Kiswahili is notoriously lax with rules of grammar, so I was having a hard time figuring out why someone with a Kenyan name spoke the way he did. Eventually, I concluded that the name may also have been Tanzanian or that he grew up there."

"Wow, that's very bizarre. And now I feel quite violated that someone got a DNA specimen from me without my knowledge."

"Oh, your DNA trail is everywhere, whatever you eat, drink, or touch. And you were in police detention for one night, so they could have gotten whatever they needed from you there. That's not surprising at all. If you're not guilty, nobody will ever find out that they took it. And if you're guilty of blowing up a building, do you think anyone is going to get hung up over why nobody asked you before taking a DNA sample from your soda glass?"

"I guess not," said Jude, his eyes going back to the printout in front of him. "So about us being related. I think that's probably the strangest of all the things that guy—Harrison or whatever his real name is—told us. I don't know anything about DNA tests, so I have no idea what a forty-seven percent similarity or overlap means, but if the guy from the lab who deals with them all the time thinks it's significant, then we're probably going to need to check it out. Even if the tests suggested we were related, how would that even work out in reality—I don't know much about my birth parents, and I'm a long way from home."

Qadir was quiet and thoughtful for a few moments, squinting his eyes in deep concentration. "There's a Swahili saying that goes, '*Ya Mungu ni mengi, huenda ikawa*,' which roughly translates to ‘God’s ways are many—anything is possible.’ I don’t know what any of this means, but if it’s true and it was meant to be, then it will come to pass.”

“OK, so what are we gonna do? I only have a few days left before I head back to Washington.”

“I have no idea,” replied Qadir, shaking his head. “I don’t even know where to begin, so we’re going to have to think about it. I’ve never really asked my uncle about my parents because I was afraid it might bring up painful memories about the war in Somalia or about how my parents died. I also didn’t want my uncle to feel I was not satisfied with all the care they took of me—both he and my aunt. Even now, I’m not sure that asking him is the right thing to do, but I’ll think about it.”

Qadir pondered this prospect for a moment before continuing. “And actually, even before this Momanyi fellow came along today, I’d been thinking of inviting you over for dinner before your departure. I’ve enjoyed interacting with you, and when I told my uncle and aunt about your misadventure, my aunt strongly suggested I invite you for a meal. You don’t have to come if you don’t want to, though my aunt will be very pleased if you accept. I had meant to ask you later in the week, but it doesn’t matter at this point. We can still plan on the dinner regardless of whether I decide to ask my uncle about what happened to my parents.”

"Sure, I'd be happy to come."

"Great! I'll talk to them and let you know more," said Qadir, rising to his feet. "Now I need to get back to work. I'll let you know the details once I confirm with them."

Chapter Twenty-Two

Doris Wilson seemed surprisingly calm and philosophical about the earth-shattering discovery when she called later that morning to chat. She didn't find the news as improbable as Jude had.

"Well, we adopted you in Minneapolis, and you may not be aware of it, but there's a large Somali immigrant population there. The only information the orphanage had about your origins was that someone left you at a safe haven baby drop-off in one of the city hospitals. We'd considered adopting a child for a couple of years, but it wasn't until I picked up a newsletter that came in the mail that I developed an odd, compelling sense of certainty that it was time to act. And the first time I walked into that orphanage and set eyes on you, I knew you were the one. I'm not afraid of what you might find in the coming days. Even if you do find your birth family—and I earnestly hope for your sake that you do—you will always be our son. If the good Lord that brought you into our lives wills it that you should find your birth family, then who am I to thwart his purposes?"

Jude had been unsure what to expect from his mother, and he found her reaction reassuring and even encouraging.

"What's Dad . . . er . . . how d'you think he'll take all this?"

Tom was already asleep when Doris called as it was about half past midnight in Clarksville.

"Your father will probably be astonished, but I'm sure he'll take it in stride. Since we don't even know if there's anything to this piece of news, I'm going to tell him it's just a possibility and nothing more."

They moved on in their conversation to more practical issues, such as his return trip home, the temporary travel documents he'd picked up from the embassy, and how he was getting by on his limited budget. By the time they were done talking, the sense of tortured uncertainty that he'd had prior to the phone call had completely dissipated. His mother had the unique ability to play down even the most dramatic and unusual bit of information and turn it into something that was merely interesting and worthy of passing mention at the dinner table.

They concluded the conversation, and Jude replaced the receiver. After milling around distractedly in his room, he decided to take a stroll downtown. In recent days, he'd grown more confident getting around in the city, with his fear of getting lost or being unable to communicate with the locals rapidly fading.

"You're going for a walk, Mr. Wilson?" called out Anyango, the receptionist, as he walked past the main desk. She had an irrepressibly jovial mien and a rather sly and nimble sense of humor. After several pleasant interactions with her in the course of his stay, Jude had concluded that she was one of the people from the hostel he would definitely miss when he returned home. On a couple of occasions, he found himself wondering what her life would have been like had she been born in the States—with her charm and quick wit, she'd probably have been presented with many more career opportunities than her current situation accorded her. Whether or not this had ever crossed her mind, he would never know, but it was clear she was not one to let her present joy get sullied by green-eyed notions of what might have been.

"Yes, Anyango. I'm trying to take in as much of Nairobi as I can in the few days I have left."

"Make sure you check out the *nyama choma*[21] restaurant on Kimathi Street that Eunice, the other receptionist, was telling you about—it's the most popular meat joint right now in Nairobi."

---

[21] Barbecued goat meat.

"You know what? I think that's exactly what I'm going to do," Jude replied enthusiastically.

"Just make sure you stay away from the *mutura*[22] since you have a flight to catch on Friday," Anyango quipped with a cheeky grin. "I don't want you to spend your flight to America running to the bathroom."

"Got it. No 'ma-too-rah' for me. Anything else I need to avoid?"

"No, I think that's the big one—and you probably shouldn't eat too much since I heard Qadir mention he'd invited you to his home for dinner."

"Ah yes. And I've heard it's rude not to eat a good-size portion when someone invites you to their home for dinner," said Jude as he stepped out the doorway, his head still turned toward her.

She gave him a quick wink and a thumbs-up sign before turning to speak to someone who had walked up to the desk.

♒

The matatu to Eastleigh was named *Buenavista*. Just like maritime vessels, matatus had names too—especially on popular routes like the one to Eastleigh. And not only names: they usually had brilliant multicolored exteriors with clever

---

[22] Spicy goat sausage.

artwork, tinted windows, and state-of-the-art sound systems, so the booming and hissing of the hip-hop music emanating from within could be felt and heard from several cars away. Most of the trendy teens in the city were happy to wait an hour for a premier ride like *Buenavista* and would dismissively wave off the less flashy conveyances that had failed to capture the imagination of their peers.

Jude had been on another matatu earlier in his visit, but it was nothing like this. He gawked at the dimly lit, elaborate interior with plush seating that felt more like an exclusive nightclub than a means of transportation. When he tried to say something to Qadir, he couldn't hear his own voice above the music, so he gave up the endeavor. By the time they got to Eastleigh, his ears were ringing, and he found himself instinctively shouting when he started up a conversation after they alighted.

As they walked briskly through the streets, weaving among the scores of people on the sidewalk, it was evident to him that this was a part of town he'd have been terrified to come to alone for fear of being mugged. Yet following behind Qadir, who strode briskly and confidently, he felt safe. They arrived at the apartment complex and climbed the stairs to the third floor, then walked halfway down the hallway and stopped.

"This is home," Qadir said with a smile, still a little breathless from climbing up the stairs. He then knocked on the door.

A male voice said something from within, then there was some shuffling before he heard footsteps approaching. Finally, the door opened, and a slender bearded man wearing an embroidered cloth cap appeared. It was Hussein.

"Aabo . . . ," began Qadir before his voice trailed off.

Hussein's gaze had turned from his nephew to Jude, and he let out an involuntary gasp. *"Subhanallah!"*[23] he said hoarsely as the tin mug he'd been holding fell out of his hand and landed noisily on the floor, splashing what was left of his tea where they stood, with some of it spraying their shoes.

"Aabo!" Qadir shouted and quickly grabbed his uncle, whose knees looked as if they were about to buckle. Jude didn't understand what was said next, as it was all in Somali, but he could see that the conversation was animated as Qadir guided his uncle to the nearest armchair in the living room and made him sit down. All this time, Hussein's gaze kept coming back to Jude, and he kept muttering wordlessly to himself. Mariam, who had been in the kitchen, heard the clamor and came out to see what it was all about. She stopped dead in her tracks when her eyes met Jude's.

---

[23] "Praise be to God!"

"*Mashallah!*[24] Yassin?" she exclaimed.

There was an extremely spirited exchange in Somali, and Jude sat in perplexed patience, wondering what was going on. Hussein and Mariam cast frequent glances in his direction, and it was clear they were talking about him. Hussein's voice was choking, and his eyes were glimmering with tears. Then the conversation began to slow down, and the tone lightened as Hussein explained something to Qadir, with Qadir stopping him intermittently to seek clarification. Finally, Qadir nodded and turned to Jude.

"OK, Jude, sorry to keep you waiting—there was a long explanation that I was trying to understand. We don't need a DNA test. The reason my aunt and uncle reacted so strangely is because you look exactly like our dad, who died many years ago. I hadn't told them anything about the DNA result, but the minute each one of them saw you, they literally thought you were a ghost. Our dad, Yassin, brought you, me, and our mother to stay here just as the war was breaking out in Somalia. My uncle and his family had been living in Nairobi for years. Unfortunately, our dad got very sick and died soon after we arrived, leaving our mom with the two of us. I'm three years older than you, and you were just a baby when we got here. Just as the extended family was trying to figure out what

---

[24] An exclamation of wonderment.

to do about our mom—who was now a young widow with no means to raise her boys—there was another family in this building with a pregnant woman who unfortunately developed complications and died in childbirth; the baby didn't survive either. That family had already begun the process of immigrating to America and had an appointment with the embassy for the interview . . ."

"Ah, I see where this is going," said Jude, nodding. "So Mom took that woman's place at the interview . . ."

"Correct. And since you were only a few months older than the other woman's baby would have been, they figured she would take you. So they got married, and Mom went for the interview as Mrs. Abdirahman, with you, Mr. Abdirahman, and his two older sons. Everything seemed to have worked well, and the plan was to figure out a way to get me there to join them afterward, once they'd settled in. Everyone thought that because it had been such a perfect coincidence, it was meant to be, and they figured our mother would find a better life for us in America. That's where things got a little complicated, and my aunt and uncle don't know exactly what happened.

"The Abdirahman family—which includes you—traveled to Minneapolis and settled there. My uncle says they initially kept in touch, with Mr. Abdirahman calling every couple of weeks or so, but before long, it became evident that things weren't going so well. He rarely let Mom—our mother's name was Amina—speak on the phone, and when she did, he was always right there, listening. My aunt suspects he was beating her, but they don't know that for a fact. Then suddenly, one day, Mr. Abdirahman called and said our mother had run away with you, and in the weeks that followed, they were unable to find you. My uncle doesn't know how much to believe of Mr. Abdirahman's story because by that time they didn't really trust him—in fact, my uncle says all these years he felt that it was possible that Mr. Abdirahman might have even murdered you both."

Hussein cleared his throat and asked a question for Qadir to translate.

"He's asking how your mother is."

Jude had started to speak, then realized what it really was that Hussein wanted to know. He shook his head somberly.

"Tell him I was raised by a *mzungu* lady—she adopted me when I was a baby, and she's the only mother I've ever known. I don't know what happened to our mother."

Qadir conveyed this information, and the expectant looks that had formed on Hussein and Mariam's faces were quickly replaced by thinly veiled disappointment. An awkward pause followed.

"What's my Somali name, by the way?" Jude asked, breaking the silence.

Hussein seemed to have understood and didn't wait for Qadir to finish translating the question.

"Warsame."

"Hmm . . . what does it mean?"

As Qadir repeated the question in Somali, a big grin unexpectedly appeared on Hussein's face, and he let out a chuckle. Mariam also broke into a smile and started shaking her head incredulously. Qadir initially seemed to have missed whatever it was that had lightened their mood, but it gradually dawned on him, and he turned to Jude. "It means 'bearer of good news.' Aabo says you proved true to your name today."

As Jude began to nod, his uncle turned to him with an outstretched hand and said, in broken English, "Welcome. You have find your way home, Warsame."

About the Author

Ndirangu Githaiga was born in Kenya and immigrated to the United States. He is a physician based in Virginia, with a passion for storytelling and the written word. His other published novels include *The People of Ostrich Mountain* (2020) and *Ten Thousand Rocks* (2021). To learn more, visit www.ndirangugithaiga.com.

Follow Ndirangu on social media at:
https://www.facebook.com/NdiranguG
https://www.instagram.com/ndirangu.githaiga/

Acknowledgements

My heartfelt gratitude goes to my wife, Magda, and three daughters, Zahra, Imani and Makena, for your unceasing encouragement. Thanks to Nyambura Githaiga, beta reader extraordinaire, for your astute observations and feedback, and to Ciru Maye for your incredible help with logistics within the Jamhuri. Thanks also to Maitu, Jennifer, Auntie Dorcas and Mbari ya Maiko for your support, as well as my entire extended family spanning multiple continents (in particular my super-supportive cousin Wangu Mureithi). Thanks also to Mbari ya Waithaka and the Muchiri family from my *gĩcagi* in Hampton Roads, especially my 'adopted' daughters Mercy Waithaka and Neema Muchiri. Thank you, Pastor Kevin Turpin, for your mentorship and practical insights on my writing journey.

Special thanks to Dr. Guled Yusuf, longtime friend and medical colleague, for your critical insights into Somali culture and language. I would also like to thank my editor, Keyren Gerlach-Burgess, as well as copyeditor, Lisa Bannick, and proofreader, Sarah Vostok, for your brilliant input and amazing attention to detail—what a team! And thanks to my ever-expanding network of friends and supporters in the different corners of the globe. Last, but not least, I humbly acknowledge the inspiring influence of the eternal Word, who modeled and perfected the art of packaging truth in parables.

CPSIA information can be obtained
at www.ICGtesting.com
Printed in the USA
BVHW092119150922
646957BV00001B/44